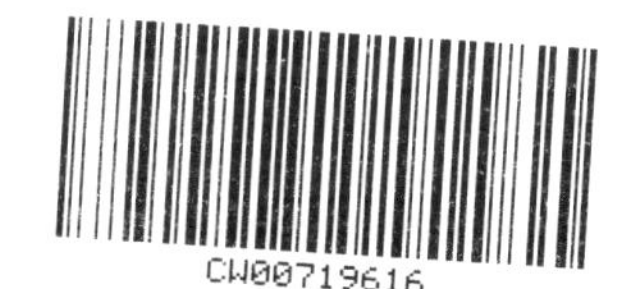

PUBLISHING DETAILS

PUBLISHER : WELLNESS AUSTRALIA PTY LTD
33 KIRWAN ST, FLOREAT PARK
WESTERN AUSTRALIA, 6014

UK DISTRIBUTOR : FITNESS LEADER NETWORK
HIGH BARN
WARNFORD
HAMPSHIRE S032 3LD
TELEPHONE / FAX : (01730) 829633

ISBN 1 875139 03 6
REPRINTED 1989, 1991, 1992, 1994, 1996

Dear Reader,

EXERCISE DANGER has been written in response to the hundreds of questions we are asked every year by coaches, teachers, fitness leaders, doctors, physiotherapists, athletes and aerobic participants regarding the relative dangers of specific exercises.

Such questions have arisen because the Western world is in the early stages of a fitness boom, that will engulf the majority of our population in the next 20 years.

Consequently, more injuries are occurring as the spread of safety knowledge fails to keep pace with the proliferation of enthusiastic participation.

Many coaches, teachers, community fitness leaders, and the media are poorly trained, and are often responsible for promoting some extremely dangerous exercises.

This situation is improving with time but not fast enough to save many thousands of people from suffering unnecessary injury.

We accept that many dynamic sports carry the inherent risk of injury, and we are culturally willing to take these risks for the pleasure that sport offers athletes and spectators alike. But **UNDER NO CIRCUMSTANCES** should any dangerous exercises be included in the **FITNESS** training programmes of the athlete, or the community fitness participant.

EXERCISE DANGER will alert you to some of the major dangers you will encounter on the road to health and fitness. Avoid these dangers and your exercise programme should be fun, effective and injury free.

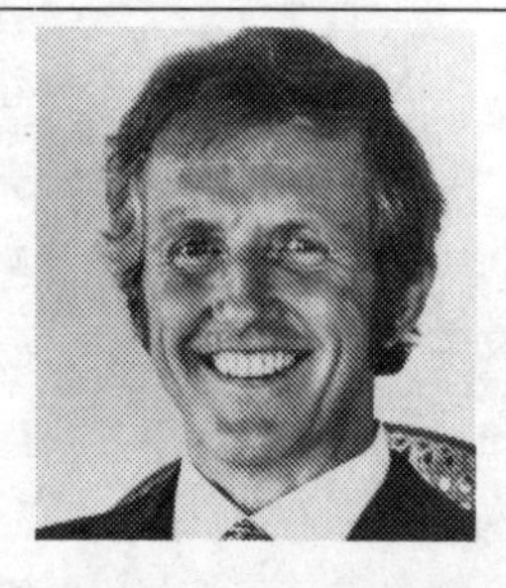

AN INTRODUCTION TO EXERCISE DANGER

by

Donald B. Ardell, Ph.D.
Director of Campus Wellness Centre
University of Central Florida

EXERCISE DANGER is a unique and useful book. It should be examined by everyone who exercises, which SHOULD be everybody. Even those who do not exercise should read it, since they are likely to realize, finally, how important strength, range of movement and endurance are to a successful life from the commentaries in **EXERCISE DANGER.**

Why stretch for mobility and flexibility? Why lift, pull or push for strength? Why run, bike, swim or otherwise use the major muscle groups for cardio-vascular, endurance-type of exercise? The SIGNIFICANCE of exercise as well as the proper WAY to go about it are explained in this cleverly done book. It is not to be missed, even by fitness experts such as aerobics instructors, who will almost surely find that a favorite routine violates some overlooked principle.

EXERCISE DANGER offers photos of exercises that are dangerous along with a discussion of why each is hazardous. Most significantly, one or more alternatives that provide the same or better benefits are suggested — and illustrated. You won't have to GIVE UP any of your favourite routines altogether, you will just want to MODIFY and IMPROVE UPON them.

EXERCISE DANGER contains more than a series of "no no's" and alternatives. It is enriched with an invaluable discussion of safety principles, a statement of exercise philosophy, a self-test prior to exercise, glossary of terms, discussion of the spine and a resource list. Those with special problems also have their special conditions addressed. For those who plan to exercise — which should be everybody, this book is a must.

CONTENTS

SAFETY PRINCIPLES

This book contains many safety principles you need to consider before exercising. The number one safety principle is to ask questions and educate yourself.

THE QUESTIONS

Every exercise included in your fitness programme should be there for a reason.

Running, walking, cycling, dancing and swimming activities for cardio-respiratory — aerobic — heart-lung (these terms all mean the same thing) conditioning and body fat reduction.

Push-ups, sit-ups, leg lifts and weight routines for toning, strength and muscle endurance.

Stretching for increased flexibility and mobility.

At a more micro level, every specific exercise you include in your programme should have a purpose.

There are three questions you should ask before including an exercise in your workout.

1. **WHY AM I DOING THIS EXERCISE?**
   Is it to strengthen or stretch a particular muscle group? Is it for cardio-vascular improvement? Is it a transition exercise to take you safely from one exercise to the next? Is it just for variety and fun but has no specific fitness purpose?
2. **IS THE EXERCISE POTENTIALLY DANGEROUS?**
   Is there any possibility **at all** that the exercise may damage your spine, tear muscles, tendons and ligaments, break bones or inflame other physical conditions?
3. **IF YES, IS THERE A SAFER AND MORE EFFECTIVE ALTERNATIVE?**

THE PHILOSOPHY

The general purpose of exercising is to improve specific components of your fitness — so that your heart and lungs function well, you avoid carrying too much body fat, your spine and joints are flexible and mobile, and your muscles are toned, strong and have a good endurance capacity.

Exercising also develops your mental fitness, increasing your self confidence and improving your self-esteem.

Each component of fitness is easy to achieve with a gentle, regular and well balanced exercise programme. But many people never achieve their desired fitness level because they fail to exercise regularly — every second day, every week, every year of their life.

Instead, most follow the "stop-start" method where long periods of inactivity are punctuated by short, fervent flurries of "crash" exercising.

Guilt ridden, they bend, kick, run and jump at a furious pace, desperate to regain their former fitness levels and eager to store for the future.

Unfortunately, the body cannot store fitness. When you stop, your fitness levels diminish rapidly.

"Crash" exercising is extremely dangerous. Whether you are an athlete, or a person exercising for general life fitness, the principles and philosophy are the same. Start **SLOWLY,** increase the intensity **GRADUALLY,** ensure their is a **SPECIFIC** reason for every exercise you include, workout **REGULARLY,** ensure your programme is more **QUALITY** than quantity, and never include any "dangerous exercises".

THE TEST

Once you have mentally committed yourself to regular physical activity, you need to assess your state of physical readiness.

You may decide that you need a complete medical check-up and will present yourself at one of the modern testing facilities, or you may wish to start immediately and take a calculated risk that all will be okay.

As a minimum requirement, check the list below for any physical conditions which may impair your physical activity.

If you answer **YES** to any of these questions, then you must receive a medical clearance before beginning any fitness programme.

1. Have you ever had any heart problems? _____
2. Do you frequently have chest pain? _____
3. Do you ever faint or feel dizzy? _____
4. Do you have high blood pressure? _____
5. Are you carrying any injuries? _____
6. Do you have arthritis or joint pain? _____
7. Do you suffer from osteoporosis? _____
8. Are you on any medication? _____
9. Are you diabetic, asthmatic or epileptic? _____
10. Are you extremely overweight? _____
11. Have you been a heavy smoker? _____
12. Are you unaccustomed to vigorous activity? _____
13. Does your family have a history of earlv death by stroke or heart disease? _____
14. Are you pregnant? _____

GLOSSARY OF TERMS

The following pages contain a series of technical terms which may be foreign to those people who are without human anatomy and physiology backgrounds.

The general meaning of each term is as follows:

Flexion	—	Bending at a joint to reduce the angle between two body parts.
Extension	—	Increasing the angle between two body parts.
Lordosis	—	Excessive and chronic arching of the lumbar spine.
Spinal Hyperextension	—	Extreme backarching of the spine.
Spinal Hyperflexion	—	Extreme forward bending of the spine.
Abduction	—	Moving arms or legs away from the body midline.
Adduction	—	Bringing arms or legs back towards the body.
Ligaments	—	Fibrous tissue bands attaching bone to bone.
Tendons	—	Collagenous fibre attaching muscle to bone.
Vertebrae	—	Series of small bones forming the spine.
Intervertebral Discs	—	Resilient cushions between the vertebrae.
Longitudinal Ligaments	—	Hold the vertebrae in place. The anterior band is strong and limits extension. The posterior band is not as strong and permits flexion.
Abdominals	—	Four layers of tummy muscles.
Gluteals	—	Muscles forming your bottom.
Quadriceps	—	The muscle group at the front of your thigh.
Hamstrings	—	The muscle group at the back of your thigh.
Ilio-psoas	—	Hip flexing muscle group attaching from your lower spine, through your pelvis to your upper thigh.

SPINAL CARE

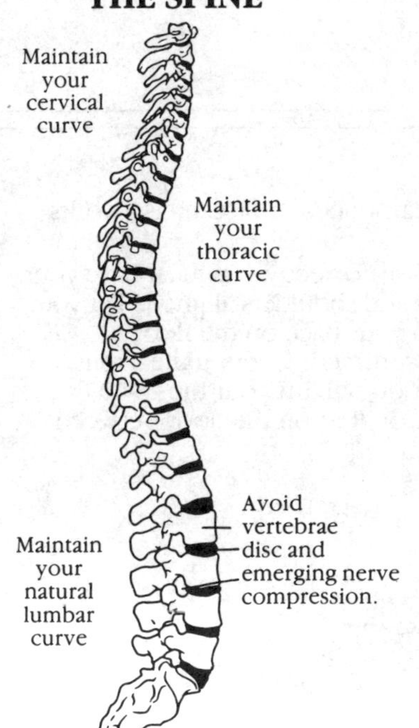

The spine is the most important structure in your body.

Dangerous exercising will put the spine under enormous pressure and damage will occur.

Fractured or dislocated vertebrae, sprained longitudinal ligaments, compressed discs, pinched nerves, torn muscles and loss of shape are only some of the problems which may arise.

Just sitting incorrectly in a chair will also cause damage and chronic pain may develop.

Your exercise programme should include exercises which strengthen the spine's supporting muscles, increase spinal mobility and help to maintain the normal spinal curves throughout life.

Don't slouch, make sure you maintain a good posture and never do any of the dangerous exercises included in this book.

Develop good lifting techniques.

DANGER

POOR POSTURE

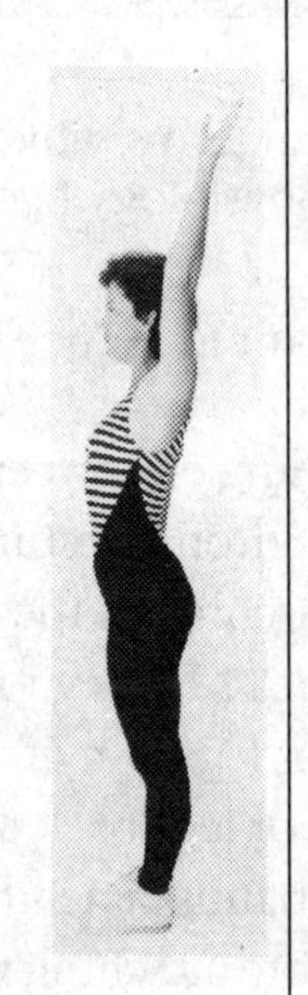

Avoid excessive arching/hyperextension of your lower back. In posture terms, this condition is known as Lordosis and is associated with weak abdominal muscles, strong hip flexors and very tight lower back extensor muscles.

This posture is often seen in pregnant women, gymnasts, women wearing high heels and people with bulging tummies.

Extreme Lordosis compresses your intervertebral discs and blocks the emerging nerve supply. Forward curving spines are equally as dangerous.

Balanced abdominal and lower back strength, plus good spinal mobility are a must. Structural problems should be evaluated by your doctor, chiropractor or physiotherapist.

DANGER RATING: Very High

INCORRECT LIFTING TECHNIQUE

The most common mistake made by people lifting any object is to stand too far away from the object, and then bend forward from the lower spine.

The forces applied to the lower back during such a lift are always greater than the design strength of this region.

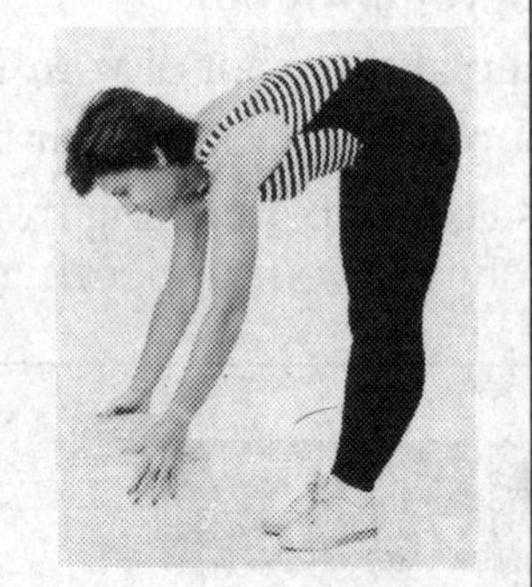

Whether it be a small, medium or large object you are lifting off the ground, you must **NEVER** bend forward at the waist with straight legs. The forces acting on your lumbar spine are often 15 to 20 times greater than would be the case if you lifted the object correctly.

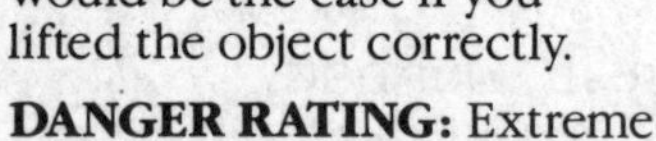

DANGER RATING: Extreme

PELVIC THRUSTS

We call this the pelvic thrust because people normally thrust their pelvis upward in a fast, repetitive manner. Their legs are usually placed wide apart, their hips often 30 or more centimetres off the ground and their back is arched. This forces weight onto the shoulders and cervical spine, and causes compression in the lumbar, thoracic and cervical vertebrae.

A very dangerous exercise with no fitness benefit. Most of the work is performed by your legs.

DANGER RATING: Very High

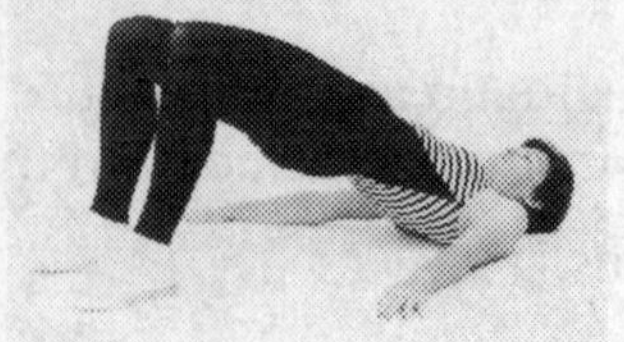

SAFE ALTERNATIVES

CORRECT POSTURE

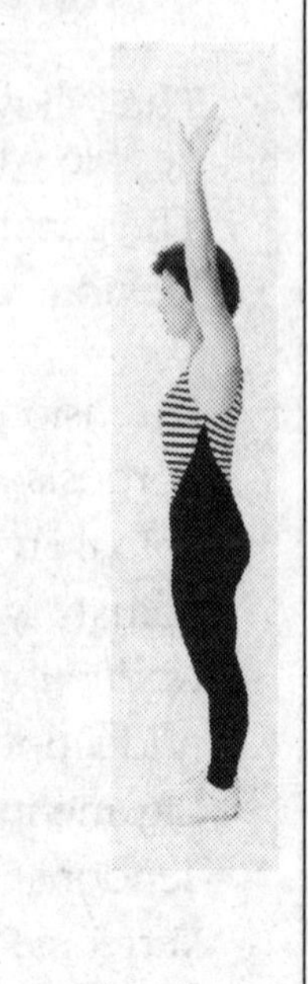

It is important to maintain a vertical alignment where the natural curves of your spine are maintained.

A strong upper-body reduces forward curving of the spine, while strong abdominals will significantly reduce Lordosis.

Avoid high heeled shoes, and avoid sagging your back when sitting. Most chairs are poorly designed and many people sit with excessive lumbar flexion.

Always try to maintain the normal lumbar curve when sitting or standing.

Your exercise programme must have a balance of abdominal and back extension work to maintain good posture and good spinal mobility.

CORRECT LIFTING TECHNIQUE

Crouch down over the object you are going to lift, with one leg forward. Flexion at each knee should not exceed about 90 degrees. Keep your body in close, your back straight and lift in the direction of your leading leg.

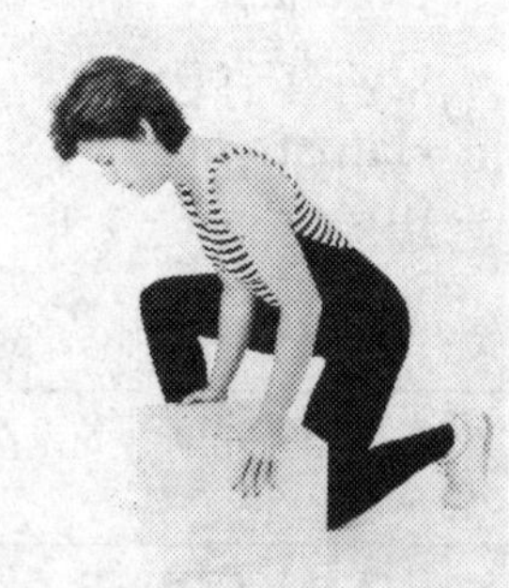

Ensure the load stays close to your body and that you grip the load firmly. If you have to hold your breath while lifting, then the load is too heavy — get someone to help or use mechanical assistance.

Keep your abdominal muscles tight and avoid any twisting actions.

PELVIC LIFTS

Often called the gluteal squeeze, this exercise works to tone your bottom.

To perform this exercise correctly you must have your feet, knees, hip joints and shoulders aligned. Tilt your pelvis under to flatten your back on the floor. Concentrate only on contracting your gluteal muscles. Isolating this contraction will lift your hips 8-10 centimetres off the floor. Rest on the floor between each repetition.

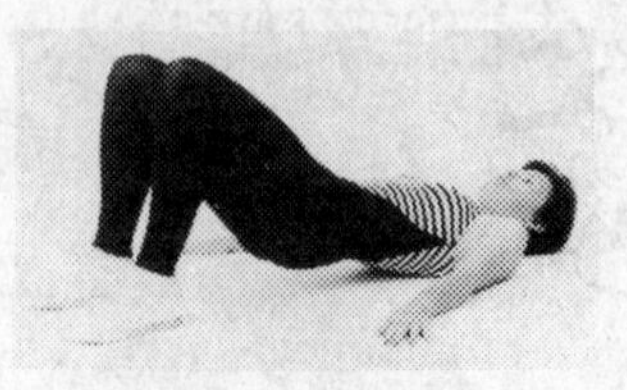

DANGER

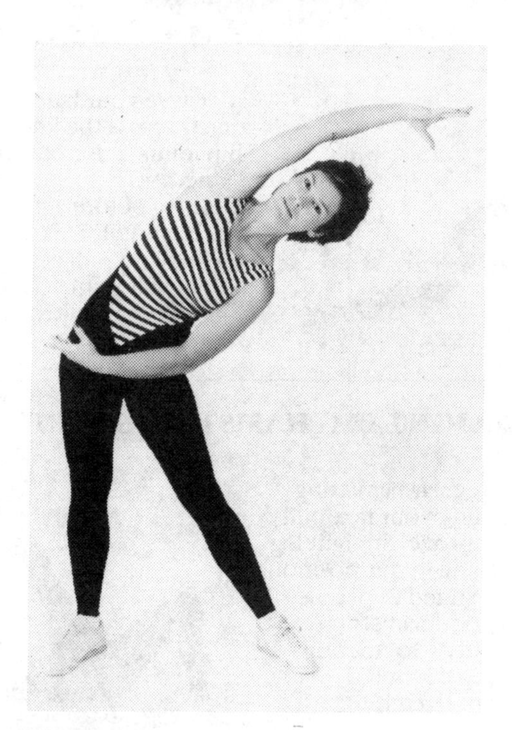

STANDING SIDE-BEND

The standing side-stretch should be one of the first exercises eliminated from your programme.

Your upper-body weight, combined with gravity, develops unnecessary spinal stress in the lumbar and thoracic regions.

This exercise causes disc compression, ligament and muscle stress, and closing down of the intervertebral foramen producing pressure on emerging nerves.

Continued use of this exercise may lead to chronic lower back pain or spinal injury.

The alternatives shown will give you greater muscle stretch. The "lying side-stretch" is particularly valuable because it gives you controlled and supported side flexion of the spine which assists development of spinal mobility.

DANGER RATING: Extreme

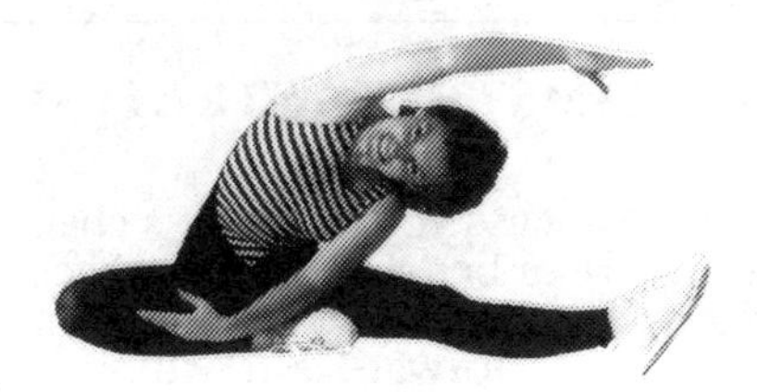

SEATED SIDE-BEND

DANGER RATING: Extreme

SAFE ALTERNATIVES

LYING SIDE-STRETCH

Move your upper-body gently to the side. Do not bend. Use the extension of your arms to gain maximum stretch. This position should allow total body relaxation and optimum stretch. It is also very good as controlled, spinal mobility work.

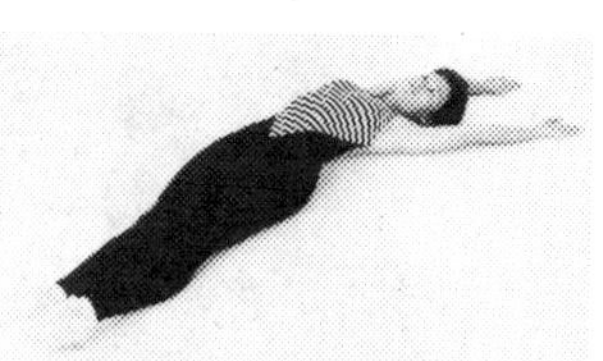

STAND AND REACH

Pretend you are reaching to pick an apple. Hold your stretch for 8-10 seconds and try to keep your spine straight. Stand on your toes to create a full body stretch.

THREE PRONG SUPPORT

This fully supported position is safe while still allowing gravity to assist the stretch.

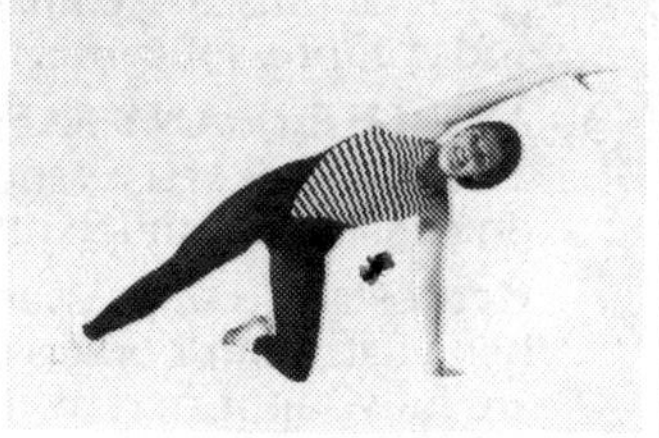

SEATED SUPPORT STRETCH

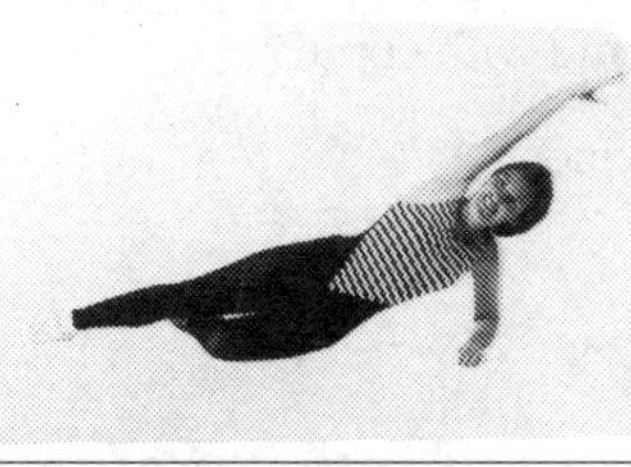

A more comfortable three pronged stretch for people with knee problems. Reach gently and hold for 8-10 secs.

KNEE SUPPORT STRETCH

This alternative is only recommended when it is impossible to work on the floor. Again, try to keep your spine straight.

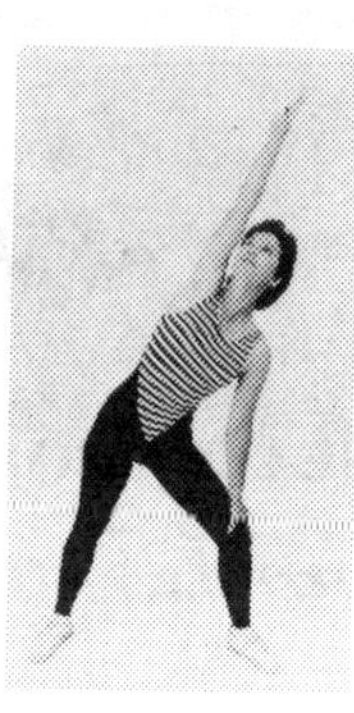

DANGER

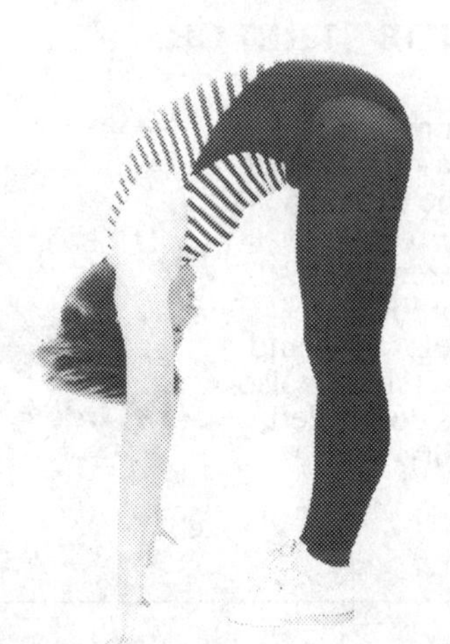

STANDING STRAIGHT-LEG TOE TOUCH

The world's most dangerous exercise!

When doing this exercise you have a perfect opportunity to ask the **THE THREE BIG QUESTIONS.**

1. **WHY AM I DOING THIS EXERCISE?**
   To stretch my hamstrings? To stretch my back? To strengthen my back?
2. **IS IT POTENTIALLY DANGEROUS?**
   Yes, I may damage my spine, and if I bounce to touch my toes, I may also tear hamstring or back extensor muscles, damage supporting ligaments, and compress the intervertebral discs.
3. **ARE THERE ANY SAFER ALTERNATIVES?**
   Yes, all the exercises shown opposite are many times safer and much more effective.

   Hydrostatic disc pressure is least when you are lying flat. Your body is totally relaxed when you are fully supported by the floor and, consequently, your stretch potential is greatly increased.

   Standing toe-touching causes total body tension rather than relaxation. Only fully relaxed muscles can be stretched safely and with control.

DANGER RATING: Extreme

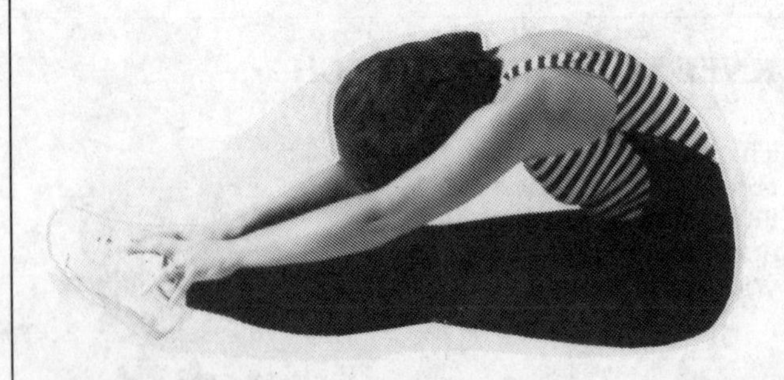

SEATED TOE TOUCH

DANGER RATING: Extreme

SAFE ALTERNATIVES

BENT LEG STRETCH

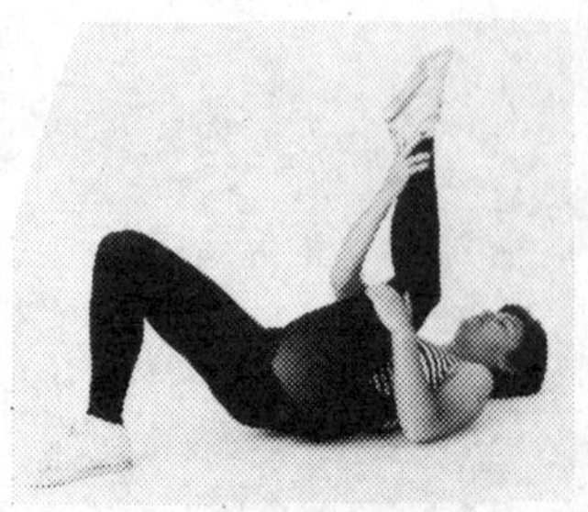

Because your hamstrings attach across the knee and hip joints, it is not usually necessary to straighten your leg before a pleasant stretch is felt. Flex fully at the hip and pull gently on your calf until you feel a mild stretch.

STRAIGHT LEG HAMSTRING STRETCH

With regular hamstring stretching your flexibility will improve. Straight leg stretching in this position is best suited to people with good hamstring flexibility. Do not pull your leg beyond a pleasant stretch.

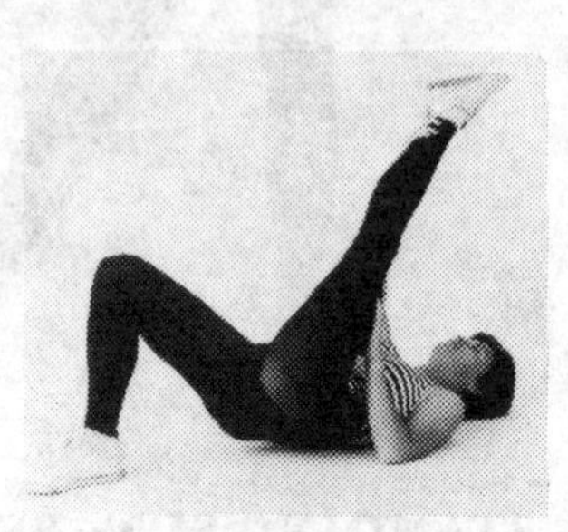

SEATED HAMSTRING STRETCH

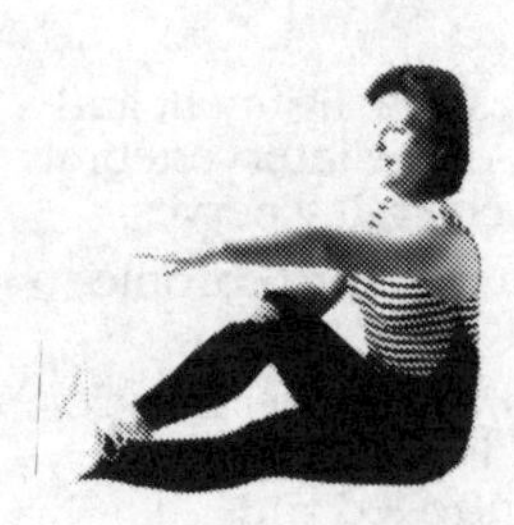

You will gain optimum stretch in this position by sitting up straight, tilting your pelvis forward, and leaning gently forward until you feel a pleasant hamstring stretch. Do not force this position. This is also good extension work for your lumbar spine.

CHAIR STRETCH

A good stretch for people with low flexibility. Place your leg on a sofa, or chair, and push up with your hands until you feel a pleasant stretch in your hamstrings.

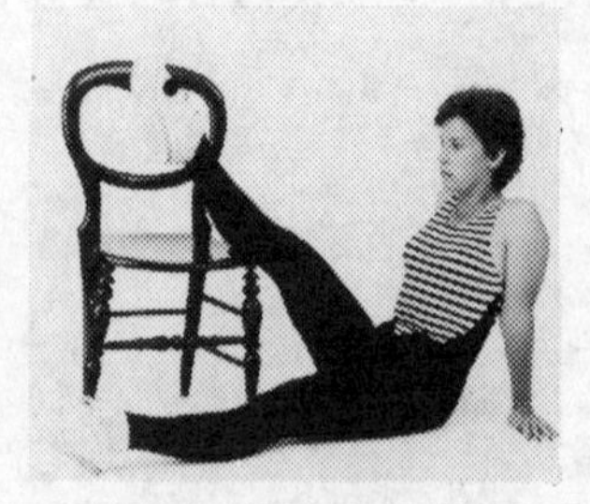

STANDING HAMSTRING STRETCH

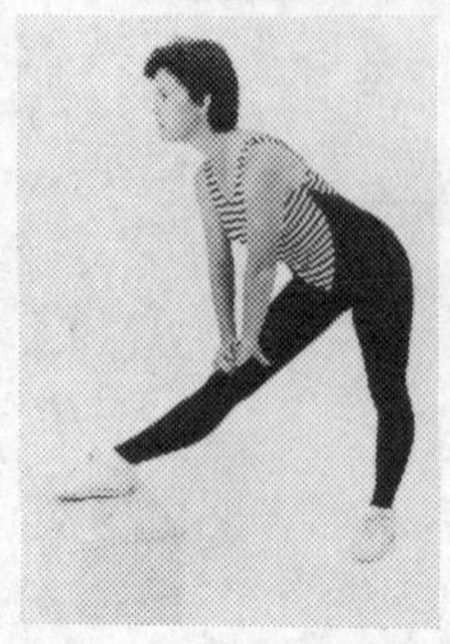

Raise your leg onto a chair or bench, keep your back straight, and support your forward lean with your hands on your knees. Bend at your hips and not in your lower back.

DANGER

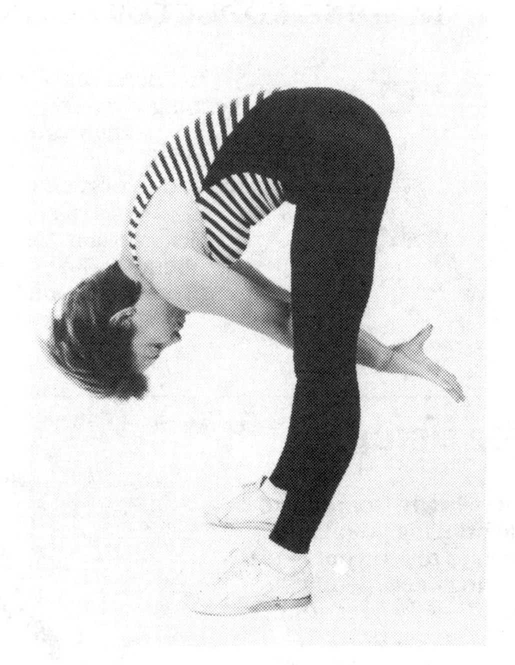

BALLISTIC PUSH-THROUGHS

As mentioned previously, all ballistic exercises are potentially dangerous. None more so than the violent stretch your gluteals, hamstrings and lower back suffer when you bounce your hands and arms through your legs.

The potential damage to emerging nerves, intervertebral discs, lower-back musculature, ligaments and vertebrae is extreme. All people, regardless of age or level of fitness, are likely to injure themselves doing ballistic push-throughs, or ballistic toe touching.

DANGER RATING: Extreme

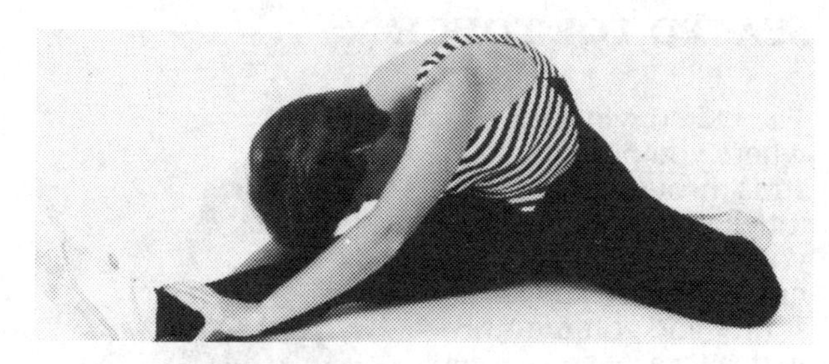

HURDLE STRETCH

Again, you are trying to stretch your hamstring muscles, but the stress on the medial ligament of your bent knee may be too great if you have a limited range of movement at the hip joint.

Remember your knee is a hinge joint which only moves in one plane — flexion & extension. If you force sideways movement you will cause stretching of the medial ligament and this may cause knee instability.

Knee instability will lead to injury during vigorous physical exercise.

DANGER RATING: High

SAFE ALTERNATIVES

ONE KNEE TO CHEST

This will stretch your gluteals. Use other stretches as shown in this book for hamstrings. Always hold the stretch and do not force past a pleasant stretch.

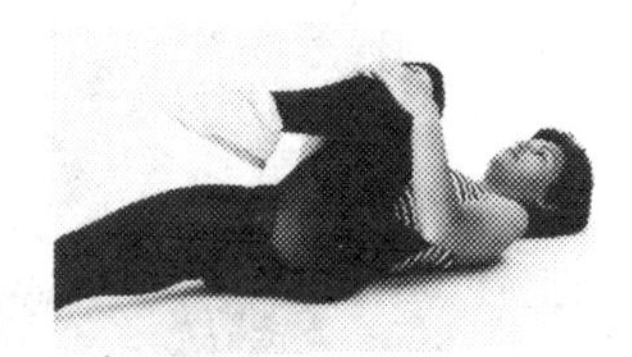

ROPE PULLING

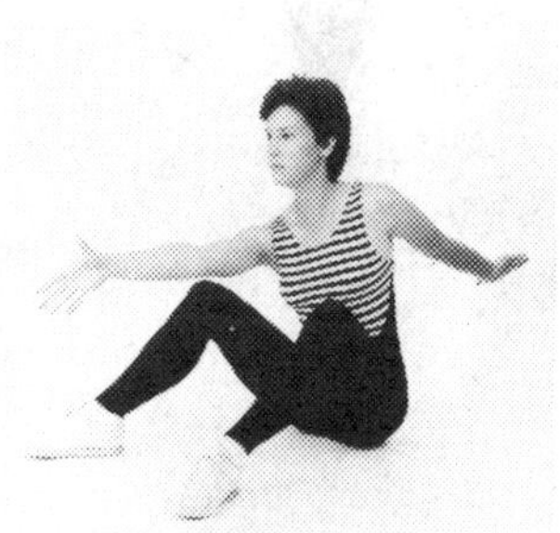

From a seated position reach forward to grab an imaginary rope. Keep your back straight and pulse from your hips — slow and continuously — alternating your arms in a reaching action. Works the arms, abdominals, and hip flexors.

SEATED STRETCH

Support your body weight with your hands, bend at the hips, keep your back straight and lean gently forward. You should feel a stretch on the inside of your straight leg, and part of your hamstrings. Hold the stretch, **DO NOT** force the position.

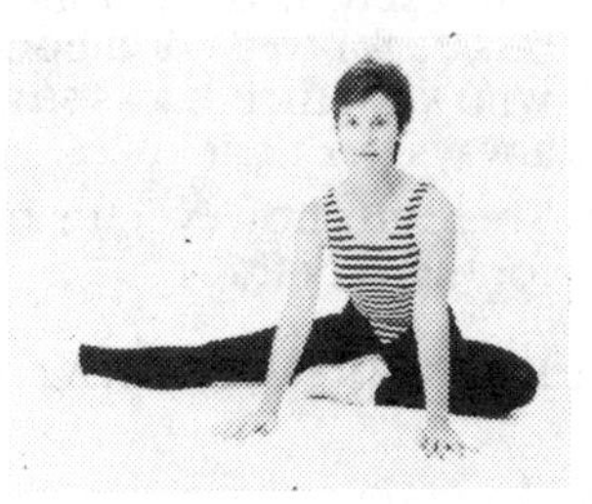

GENTLE TWIST

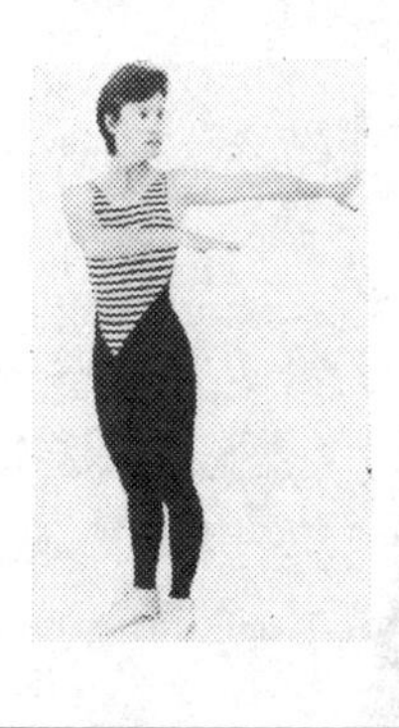

Move slowly to twist and reach to the side. This will stretch part of your shoulders, upper back and sides. **DO NOT** push past the point of a pleasant stretch. Increases lower spine mobility.

TWO KNEES TO CHEST

Pull up tightly and you will feel some stretch in the lower back and gluteal muscles. A nice stretch after any standing work. Relieves some of the spinal compression.

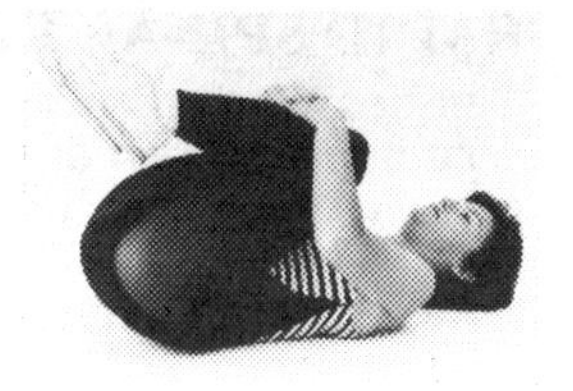

DANGER

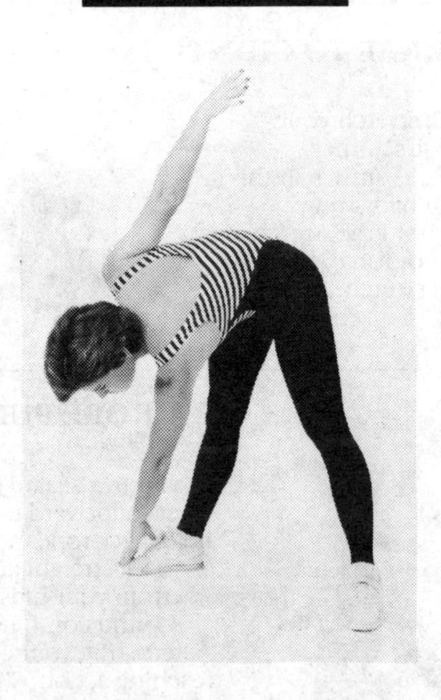

WINDMILLS

Windmills produce simultaneous twisting and forward bending of the spine.

The potential damage to structures and tissue in the lower back is very high.

This exercise is a definite **NO** for beginners, but may be safe for well conditioned, advanced participants who keep their backs straight, bend at the hips and always flex their knees.

There are, however, many safer alternatives, even for the very fit.

DANGER RATING: Very High

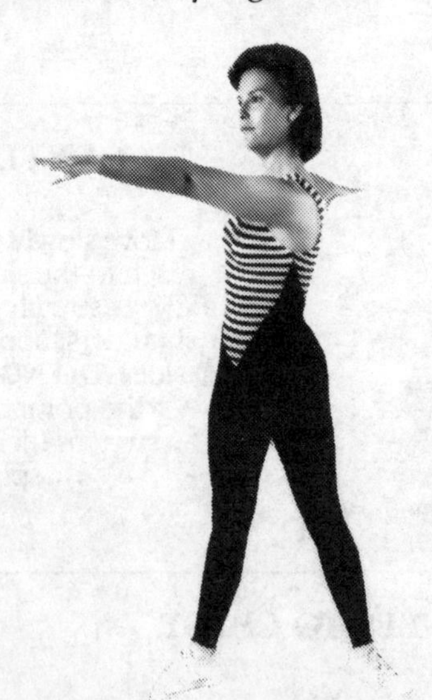

RAPID SPINAL TWISTING

Twisting your spine rapidly may severely damage your intervertebral discs. Avoid completely. All spinal rotation should be slow and controlled.

DANGER RATING: Extreme

SAFE ALTERNATIVES

STANDING ADDUCTOR STRETCH

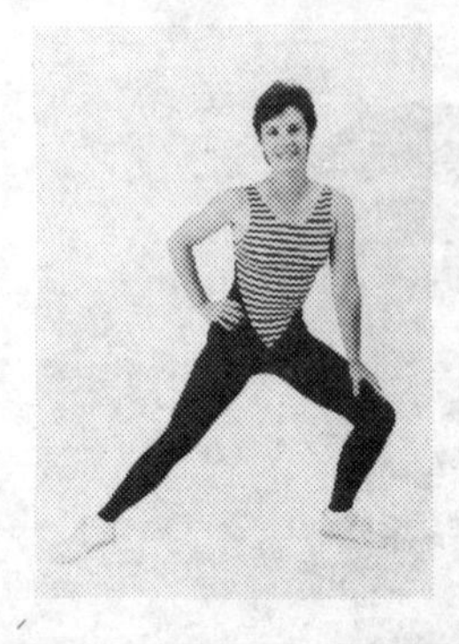

Bend one leg while keeping your opposite leg straight and facing forward. This will stretch the adductors and groin of your straight leg. Make certain your knee bends in line with the direction in which your foot is pointing.

SIDE LUNGE

Move slowly from side to side bringing your hand down to touch your bending knee. Bend your knee directly over your foot. Keep your back straight and tummy flat.

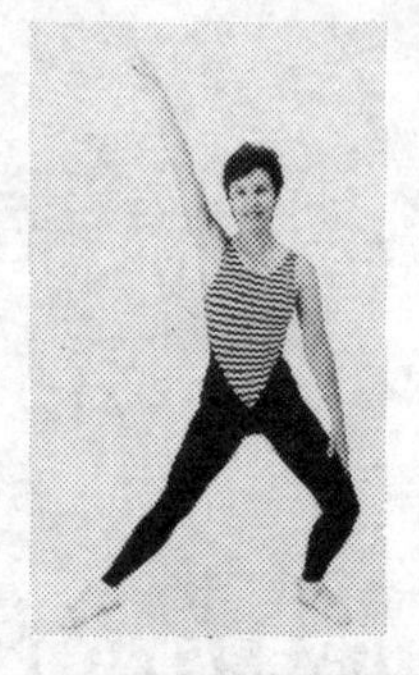

UPRIGHT WINDMILLS

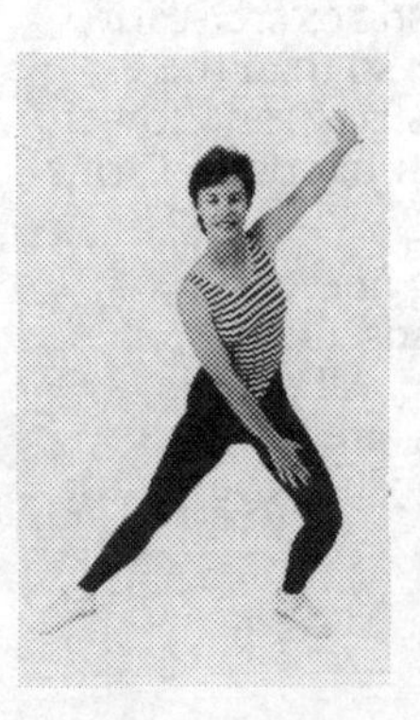

Move as per the side lunge, but this time bring your opposite hand to touch your upper leg. Again, keep your back upright and your abdominal muscles pulled in tightly. Concentrate hard on your posture and technique.

SEATED TOE TOUCH

The seated windmill where you push your arms through your legs to touch your toes. Keep your knees bent and move forward and back slowly and continuously with alternate arms. Keep your back straight.

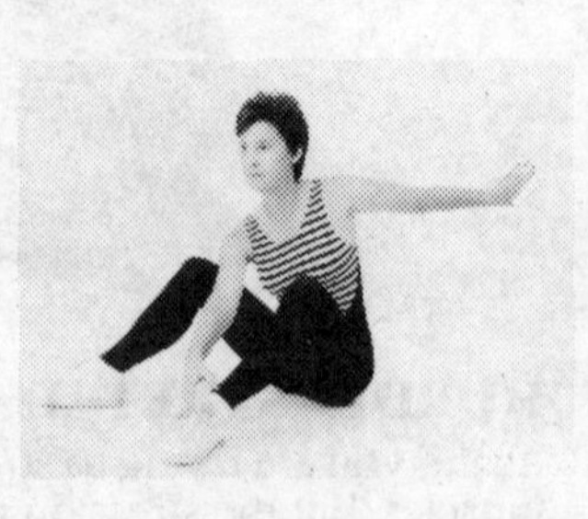

SWING & TOUCH

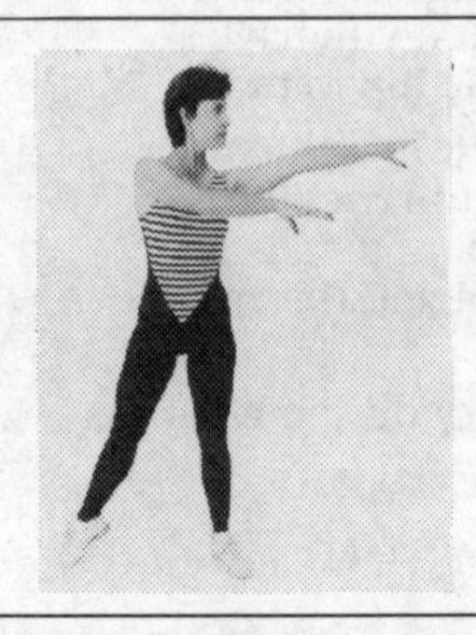

Swing your arms to one side while you step out and touch your opposite foot on the ground. A low impact, full body movement.

DANGER

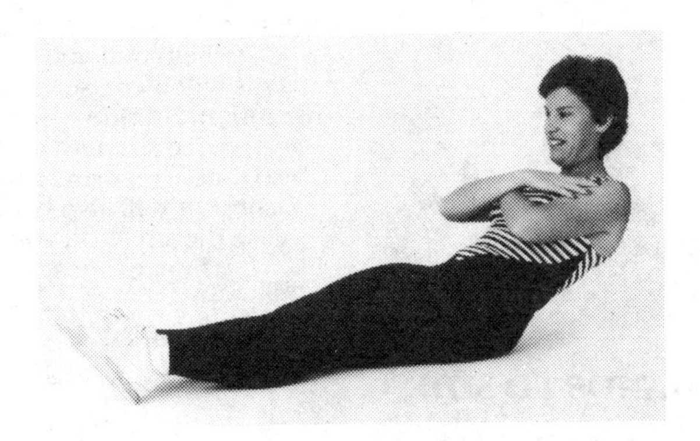

SIT-UPS WITH STRAIGHT LEGS

Strong abdominal musculature is necessary for the development of high intra-abdominal pressure (I.A.P.). Very good I.A.P. leads to strong anterior support of your torso and a more even distribution in the load carried by your spine.

Straight leg sit-ups produce only minimal abdominal strengthening. Instead, they work a group of muscles called hip flexors — Ilio-psoas muscles — which attach from your lower spine onto the top of your legs — femur.

Repeated strengthening of the hip flexors often increases lumbar arching, and causes disc and vertebral compression. Lordosis may develop.

Some strengthening of the hip flexors should be included in your programme, but **NOT** through the use of straight leg sit-ups. High knee marching, step-ups, jogging, cycling and leg raises in the water are good strengthening exercises for your hip flexors.

The "Cobra on Elbows" stretch will help lengthen your hip flexors and reduce excessive lumbar lordosis, but strong abdominal musculature will contribute most to reduced back arching.

DANGER RATING: Very High

SAFE ALTERNATIVES

BENT LEG SIT-UP

Bend your legs to a comfortable position and curl up in a slow and controlled manner. There is no need to curl-up past 45 degrees. If you do sit-up to 90 degrees, keep your back straight. The abdominal muscles do the major portion of their work in the first 30-40 degrees of the curl.

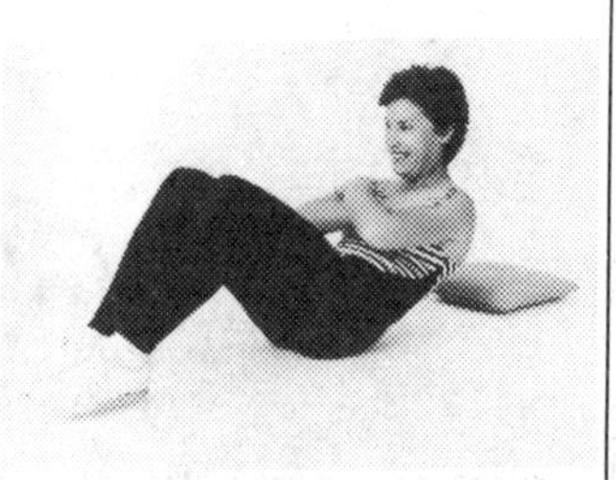

SPINAL CURL

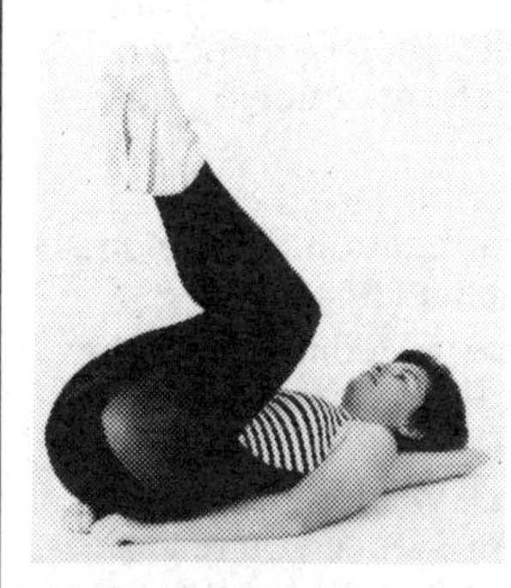

Place your hands under your buttocks, bring your knees to your chest and begin small spinal curls. Do not allow your legs to drop. The spinal curl works mainly the lower abdominal region. Keep your tummy tight and flat to avoid the development of a small bulge in the lower abdomen. Flattened tummies are a must in all abdominal exercises.

CRUNCHES

A high intensity abdominal curl, and **NOT** recommended for unconditioned people. Bend at the knees to help keep the leg weight over your body. This is particularly necessary, if you have poor hamstring flexibility, to avoid lower back stress.

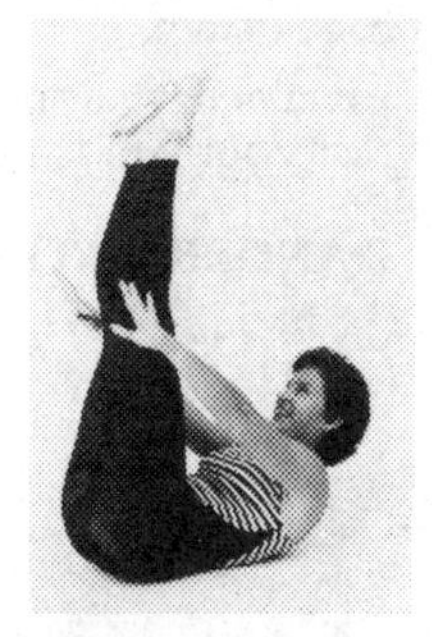

DIAGONAL CURL

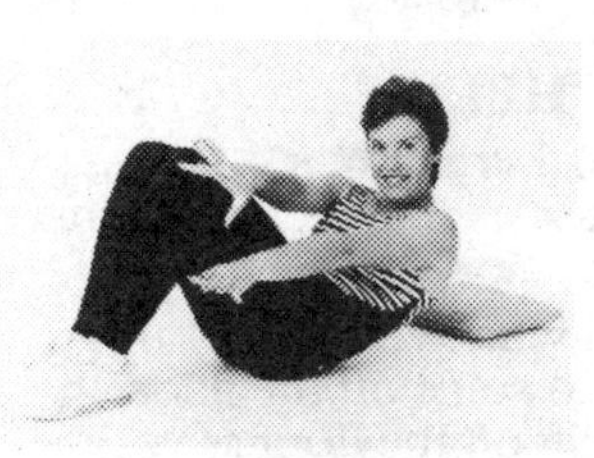

This exercise should help condition the oblique abdominal muscles. Never over twist and always do this exercise slowly. Always use a small pillow and rest between each repetition.

CHAIR CRUNCH

A low intensity abdominal crunch that can be made easier by using your hands behind your legs to help pull you up. This tones abdominal, arm and chest muscles simultaneously.

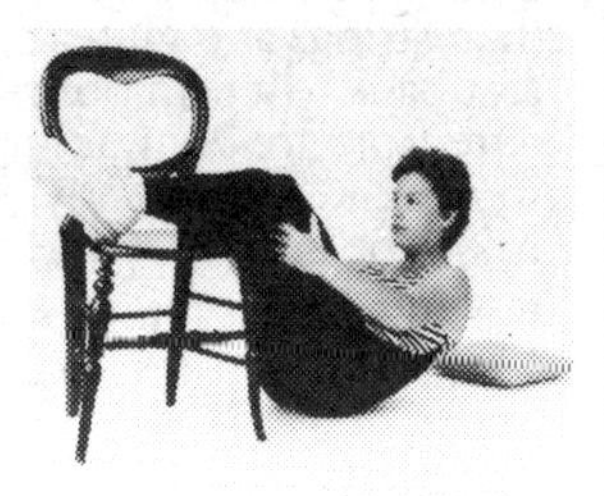

DANGER

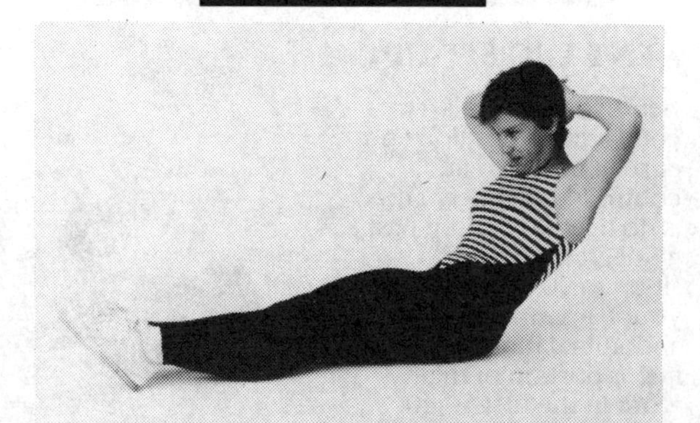

SIT-UPS WITH HANDS BEHIND HEAD

The danger in this exercise occurs when you use your hands and arms to pull yourself up, instead of allowing your abdominal muscles to do the work. Your hands pull your head forward, hyper flexing your cervical spine, compressing the intervertebral discs, and putting pressure on the emerging nerves. This may cause headaches or referred pain in your neck, arms or upper-torso.

The force with which many people jerk their heads can also lead to damage of the longitudinal ligaments which help to hold the vertebrae in place.

Your hands and arms should be placed in one of the safe alternative positions. Bend your knees up and curl-up slowly — with control.

The majority of your abdominal work is done in the first 30-40 degrees of the curl-up. Once you reach this position, roll back down and repeat the exercise.

Keep your abdominals flat, your pelvis and lower back pressed flat against the floor, and your rib cage down.

Always have a small pillow behind your head and rest your head and neck between each repetition.

DANGER RATING: Very High

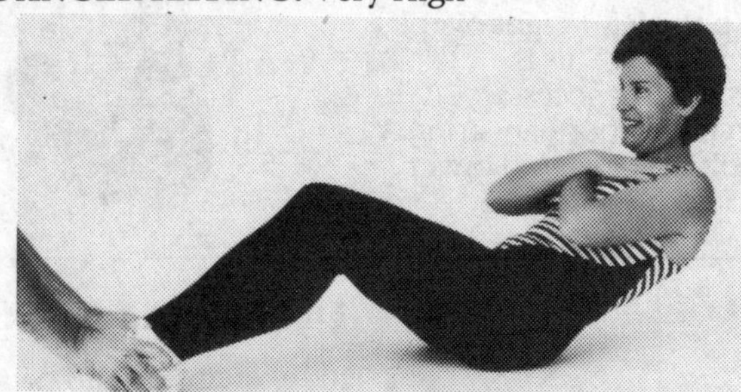

SIT-UPS WITH FEET HELD

To gain maximum abdominal strength, it is necessary to isolate the abdominal muscles and exercise them without the assistance of the hip flexors.

Hip flexor use is minimized when your knees are bent and your feet are free to come off the floor. In this position your feet will lift off the floor as you begin to curl-up. This will require your hip extensors (hamstrings and gluteals) to contract and force your feet back to a firm position on the floor. As your hip extensors are contracting, your hip flexors are forced to relax. Consequently, your abdominals are isolated to do the curl-up work.

NEVER have your feet held during sit-up exercises. This action will lessen the quality of your abdominal curl.

SAFE ALTERNATIVES

HANDS ON LEGS

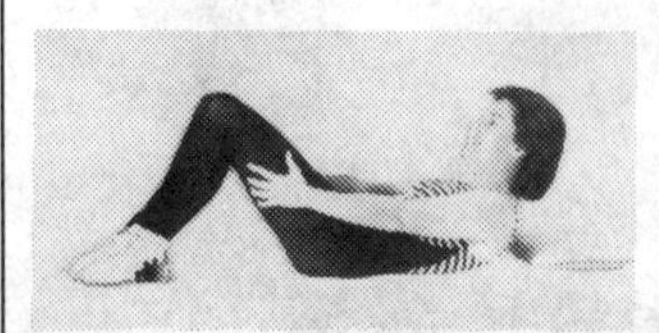

The easiest of all abdominal curls. Use your hands to help pull you up. This will increase your repetitions, improve your abdominal strength and help tone your arms and chest. It will also help ease the stress on your neck muscles.

HANDS TO SIDE

A low intensity sit-up, but slightly harder than the "hands on legs" sit-up. Keep your hands by your sides at all times. Keep your tummy flat and peel slowly off the floor.

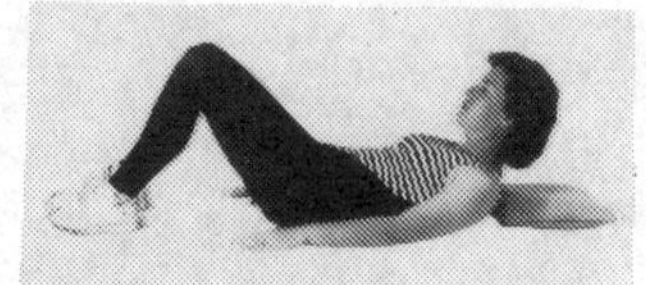

HANDS ON CHEST

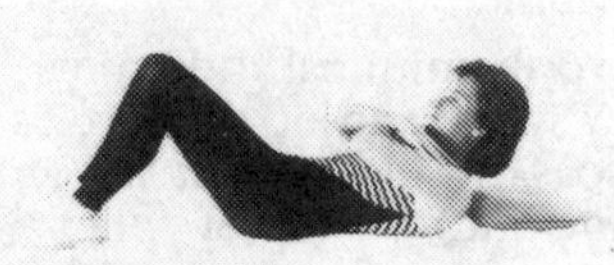

A moderate intensity sit-up, with the most common and comfortable arm postion for people of intermediate fitness. Remember to always use a small pillow.

HANDS AT EARS

A moderate to high intensity sit-up for people with advanced abdominal strength. Do not grab your ears, and avoid flinging your elbows forward. If this is too difficult, lower the intensity by moving your arms back onto your chest.

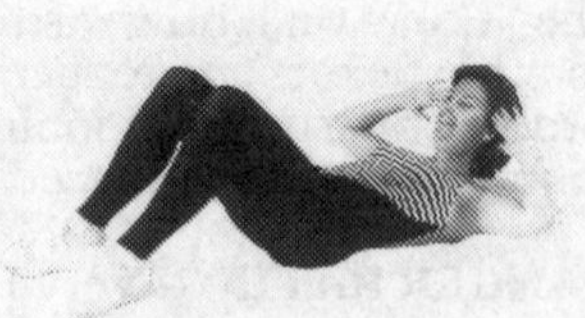

HANDS ABOVE HEAD

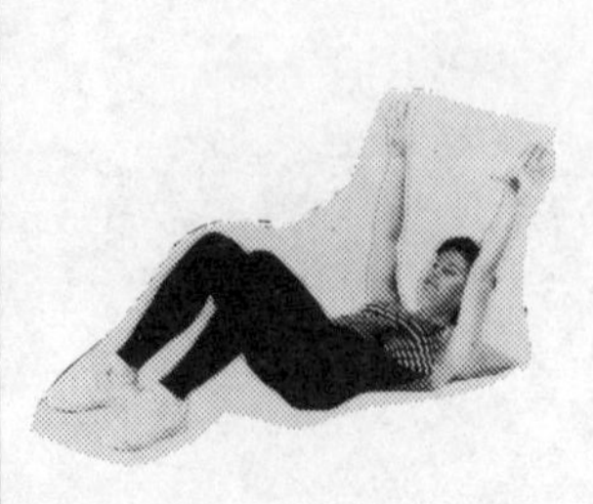

The hardest of all the conventional sit-ups. Avoid flinging your arms forward to lift yourself up. This is an advanced abdominal exercise for those with good abdominal strength. Flinging arms defeats the purpose of the exercise.

DANGER

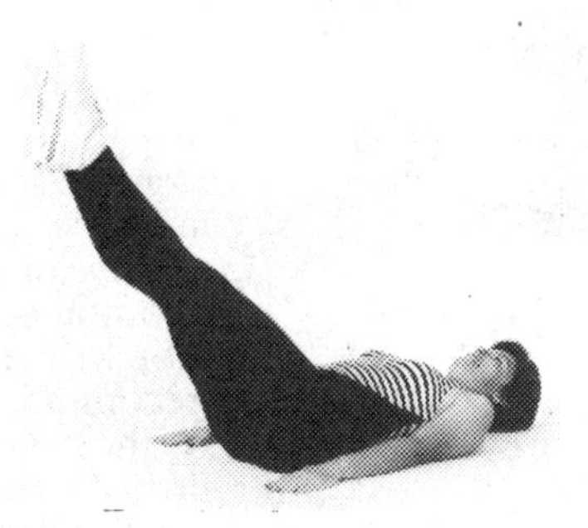

DOUBLE STRAIGHT-LEG RAISES

Double straight-leg lowering and raising works the hip flexors, but does little to strengthen your abdominal muscles.

You must remember that your abdominal muscles **DO NOT** attach onto your legs. Abdominals flex your trunk, and only isometrically contract during straight-leg raises to help reduce the pressure on your lumbar-sacral spine.

Compression injuries to your discs and vertebrae will occur. So too will muscular tears and ligament damage.

DANGER RATING: Extreme

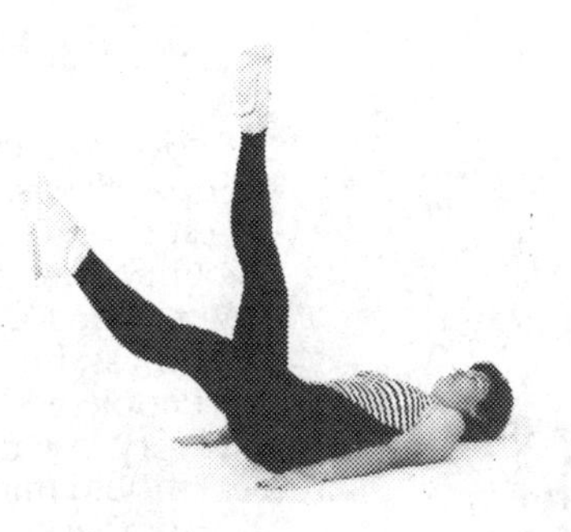

STRAIGHT-LEG SCISSORS

Sometimes done as a punishment exercise by non-thinking coaches and teachers.

These exercises are totally inappropriate for abdominal development and you should critically question anyone you see instructing people in this way.

Holding your feet and legs just off the ground is for idiots. Make sure you and your children are not doing any of these exercises.

DANGER RATING: Extreme

SAFE ALTERNATIVES

LEG CURL

Again, use your pillow to support your head. This exercise requires you to keep your knees bent at all times, and curl your legs to your chest. Good for your quadriceps and ilio-psoas muscle groups. An advanced exercise.

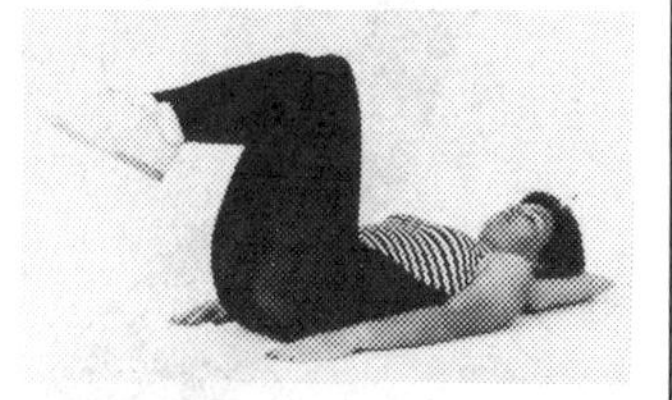

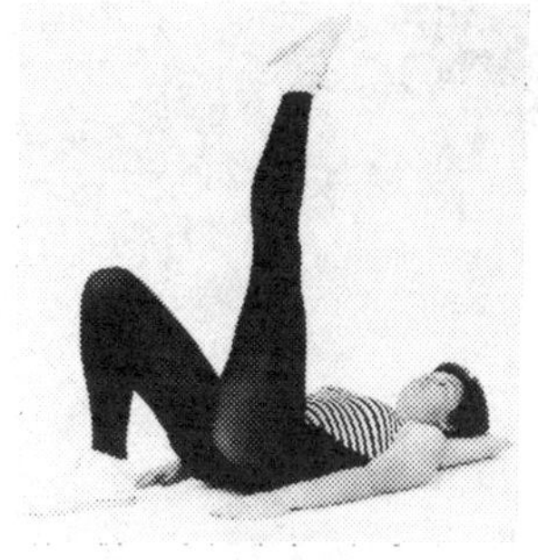

SINGLE LEG RAISES

Keeping one leg bent reduces the stress on your lower spine and back. Keep your repetitions to a minimum and avoid if you are a beginner or have heavy, fatty legs. Safe for advanced level people.

HIGH KNEE MARCHING

A high intensity, low impact exercise to strengthen your quadriceps. Marching will tone your upper thighs far quicker and safer than straight-leg raising. Keep your tummy flat and your body upright. **DO NOT** lock your knees.

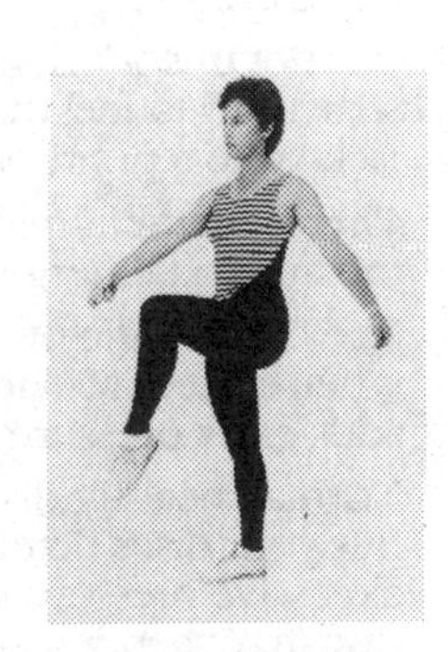

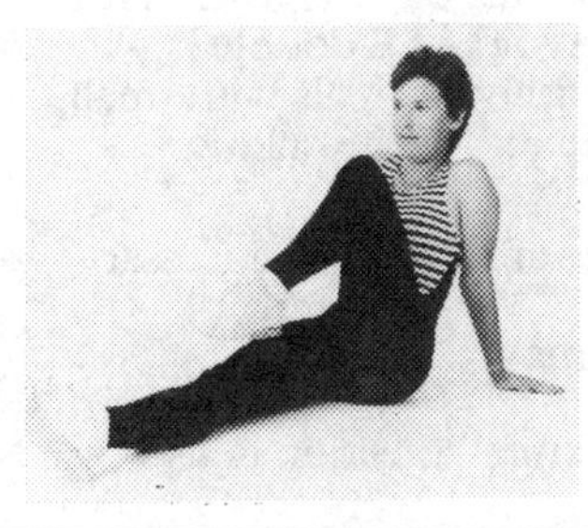

SINGLE LEG CURL

A low intensity hip flexion exercise. Keep your back straight and bring your knees to chest in alternate repetitions. Place your hands behind you for support.

SPRING KICKS

Spring off one leg and kick out the other leg. Step-kick to lower the intensity of this work. Increase the intensity by raising your kicking leg higher. Keep the support leg flexed and **DO NOT** lock your knees.

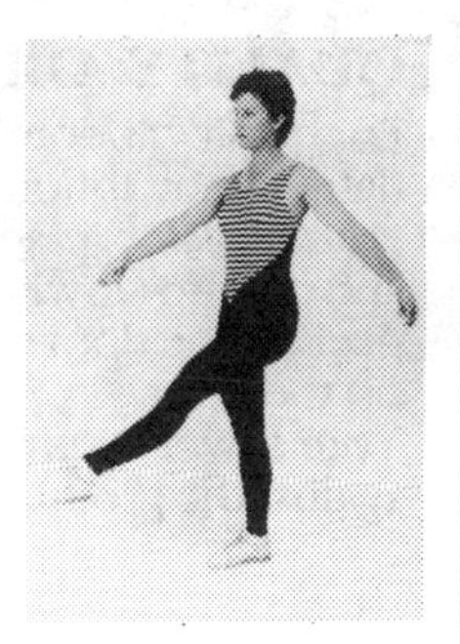

DANGER

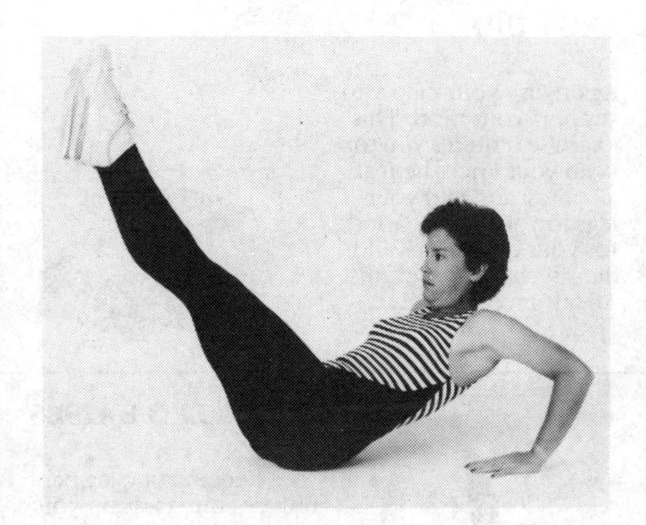

JACK-KNIFE KICKS

Like double-leg raises, jack-knife kicks will put excessive stress on your lower back and spine.

It is not uncommon for people with unstable spinal structures to feel the lumbar vertebrae moving during jack-knife repetitions.

This movement may lead to disc damage and pressure on emerging nerves.

The hydrostatic pressure in your discs is greatest when seated. Moving your legs back and forward adds extra pressure.

Normal, healthy discs will absorb the extra stress. But your discs deteriorate as you age and, if excessive pressure is applied, nuclear fluid from the disc may seep into surrounding tissues causing pain and stiffness.

This is just one of many potential back injuries. Treat your back with great care. Avoid **ALL** double leg-raising work. Develop strong abdominals with small spinal curls, and your hip-flexors with walking, jogging and bicycling exercises.

Compression relief stretches are also very necessary.

DANGER RATING: Extreme

Seated cycling in the "jack knife" position is also extremely dangerous.

QUALITY ABDOMINAL EXERCISES

For quality abdominal exercising, remember to flatten your abdominals, keep your knees bent and your feet free, place your hands in a safe position, and curl-up slowly. You should feel your vertebrae peel off the floor. Curl until your middle back is off the floor.
Your lower back should always remain pressed against the ground.

SAFE ALTERNATIVES

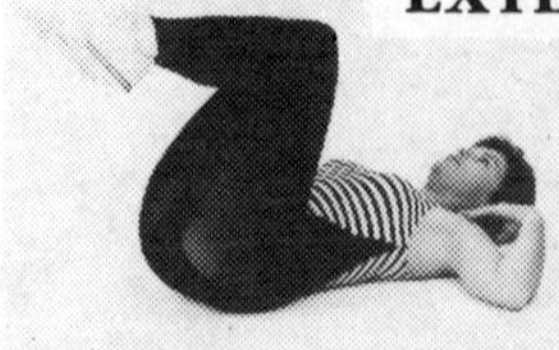

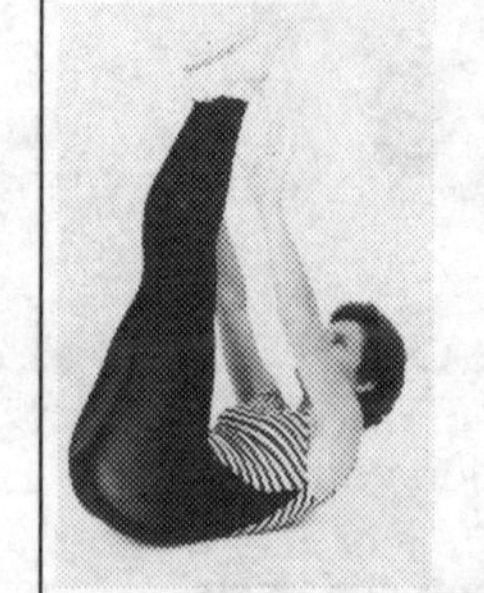

EXTEND AND CURL 1 and 2

Starting position is as shown. Your legs are then extended at the knee and you curl-up to touch your shins or feet. This is a combined quadriceps-abdominal exercise and is recommended only for those with advanced fitness levels. This is the best alternative to the jack-knife kicks.

CHAIR CURL

Make sure you have a very stable chair. Raise your legs from the floor, keeping your body weight back. Ensure your back is straight and your abdominals contracted.
A moderate intensity exercise.

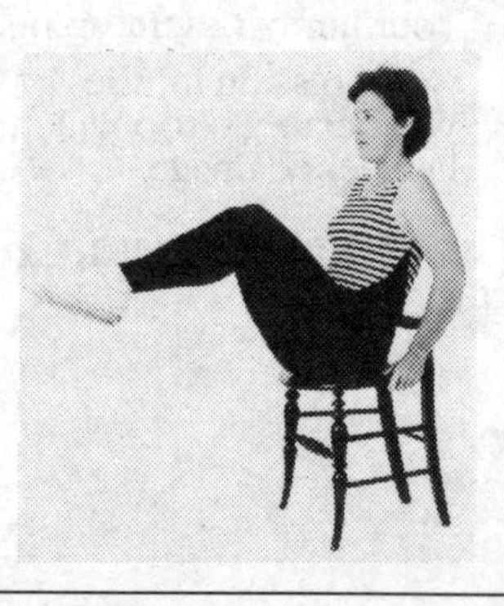

STAND AND SIT

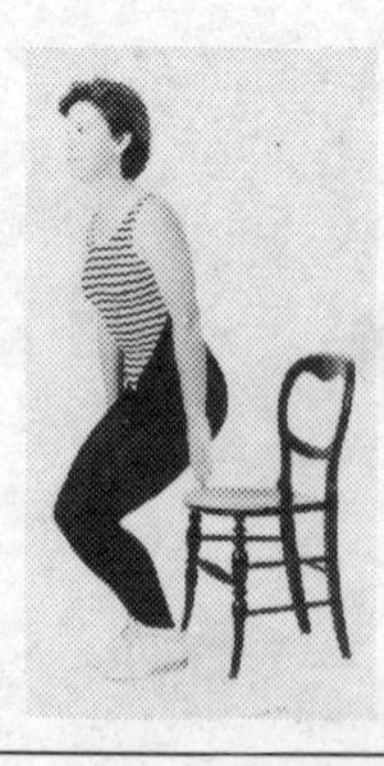

A good exercise for your quadriceps, hamstrings and, to a small degree, your abdominal muscles. Very safe for all levels of fitness, but very tiring. People with bad knees and very low fitness levels should minimize their number of repetitions.

FULL BODY STRETCH

This is a must at the end of every session where abdominal work has been done. Stretch out fully and take a deep breath.
You will feel your abdominals stretch. Helps relieve spinal compression.

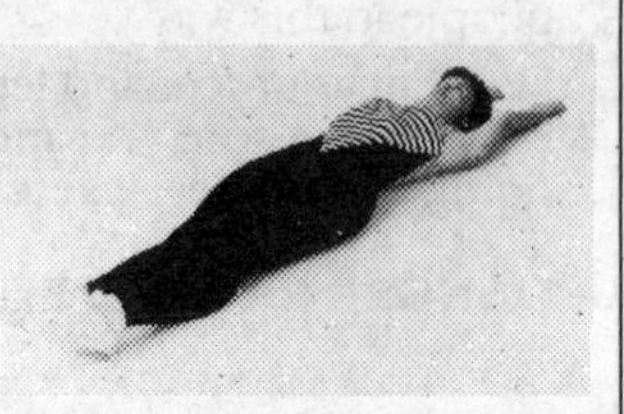

DANGER

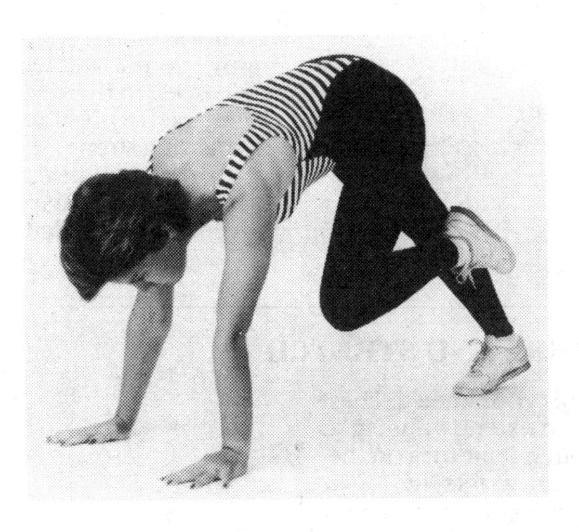

EXCESSIVE STARTS

Not a good exercise for beginners, those who are overweight, people with high blood pressure, the elderly or sufferers from R.S.I.

In fact, this exercise could be dispensed with completely and no-one would care. Besides being a transition exercise from floor work to standing position in an aerobics class, "starts" offer little other value.

By holding this position your upper-torso, neck and arm muscles are in constant isometric contraction. This leads to a build-up in blood pressure as the muscles close-down the arteries and veins in this region.

Many people also suffer wrist and elbow injuries trying to hold this position for what is often an excessively long time.

The dangers in this exercise are too great, and the discomfort people complain of is too frequent, for "starts" to be used as a regular exercise.

Give it a miss. Try the alternatives. Keep your body upright during cardiovascular work.

DANGER RATING: High

SAFE ALTERNATIVES

KNEE TO CHAIR

Use the back of your sofa, a very stable chair, or the wall to support yourself. This gives you stability, markedly reduces the pressure on your wrists and prevents the feeling of blood rushing to your head. Lift your leg up and down.

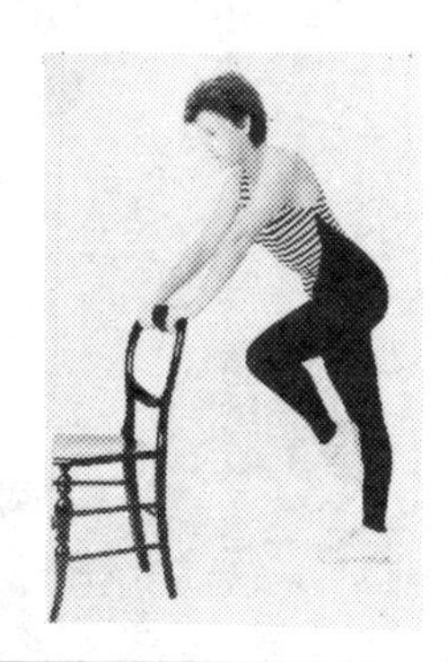

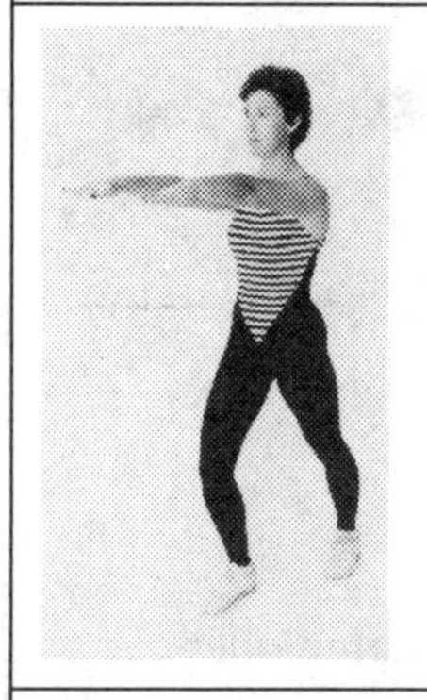

FORWARD LUNGE

Step forward and back on alternate legs. Use your arms for balance. This is a very low impact-low intensity exercise but you will feel your legs working.

KNEE LIFTS

The next three exercises offer an example of ever increasing intensity. High leg lifts increase the leg work while claps add arm work intensity.

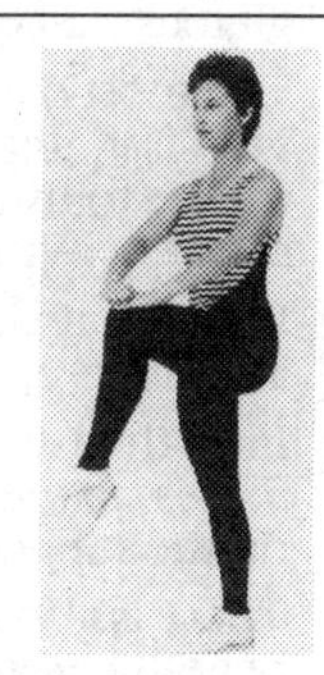

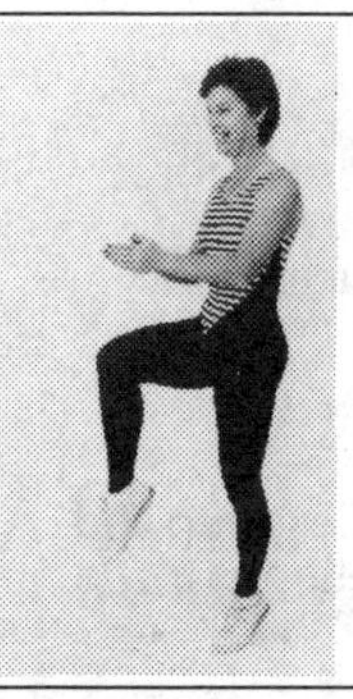

KNEE LIFT & CLAP

You may either step for low impact, or hop to increase the intensity of this work. But remember, hops will also increase the impact forces.

CLAP UNDER LEG

Notice how Jane keeps her back straight and her head upright. Always ensure you maintain good posture when exercising. Good posture and technique will drastically reduce your potential for injury.

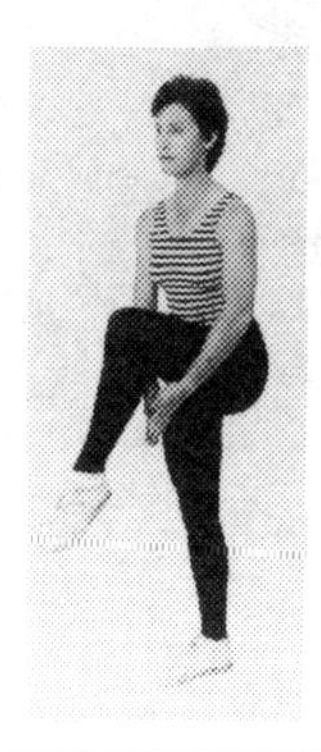

DANGER

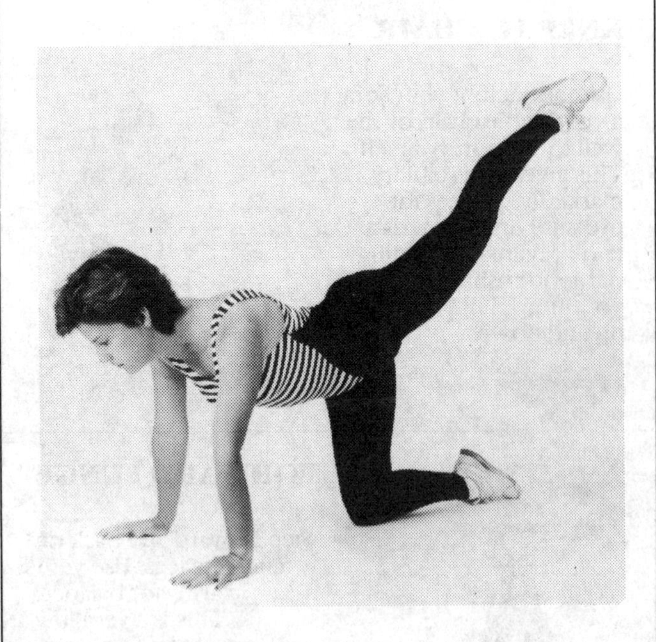

DONKEY KICKS

This exercise is designed to tone and strengthen gluteus maximus — "your bottom".

The most common problem in this exercise is the very fast, uncontrolled, ballistic movement causing the leg to fly high and your lumbar spine to arch, or severely hyperextend.

If the momentum is sufficient, the cervical spine will also hyperextend.

In both instances, there are severe compression forces on the vertebrae and discs, and severe stress on the supporting muscles and ligaments.

There is also minimal toning and strengthening benefit because the momentum reduces the gluteals' workload. Vertebral fractures or dislocation may occur.

It is also very possible during this exercise to force the hyperextension to a point where the nerve supply to your legs is momentarily reduced and severe nerve injury may occur.

NEVER do any exercise which includes **FORCED HYPEREXTENSIONS.**

Remember, the idea is to isolate a muscle group and to work it with controlled, quality repetitions for maximum toning and strengthening.

DANGER RATING: Extreme

SAFE ALTERNATIVES

HAMSTRING CURL

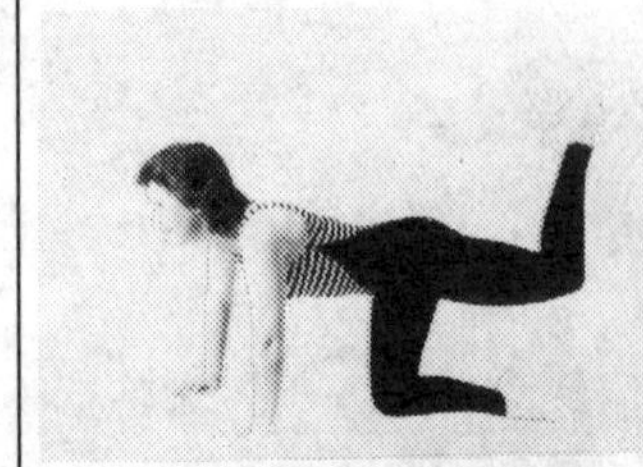

Keep your thigh horizontal and slowly move your lower leg, 90 degrees, to the vertical. repeat 8 to 16 times. A hamstring strengthening exercise. Gluteals also work. Keep the movement controlled and your back straight.

CURL AND STRETCH

Curl your knee to chest then extend your leg to touch your toes on the floor. Works the quadriceps, hamstrings and gluteals. Again, keep the movement controlled and rhythmical.
The quality of each repetition is essential. Speed is dangerous!

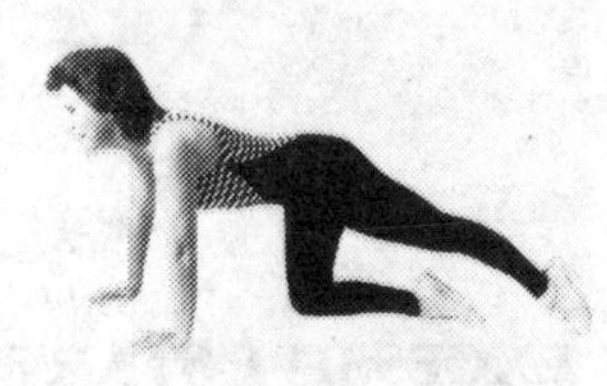

LEG LIFT

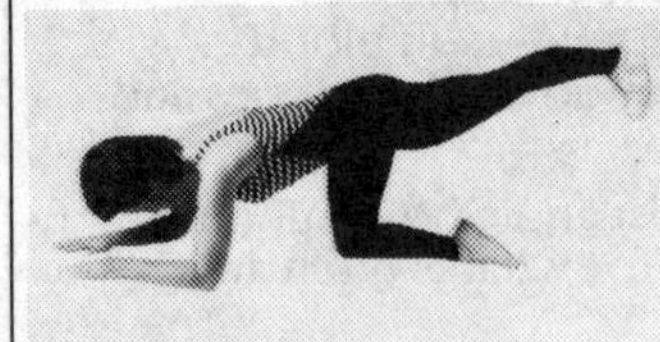

Keep your leg in line with your back. Rest your forehead on the ground (pillow), flex your foot, lead with your heel and gently pulse your leg up and down in very small movements. Excellent for hamstring, gluteal and lower back strength. People with blood pressure problems may find the head down position uncomfortable.

STEP-UP

Stepping up and down on a bench will help tone your bottom. The higher you step, the more your gluteals will strengthen. Use stairs where possible in daily life to help keep the gluteals toned.

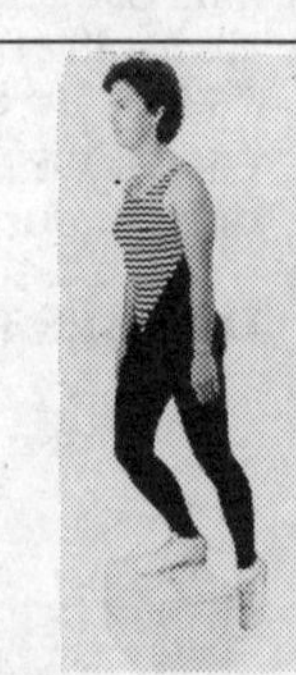

GLUTEAL STRETCH

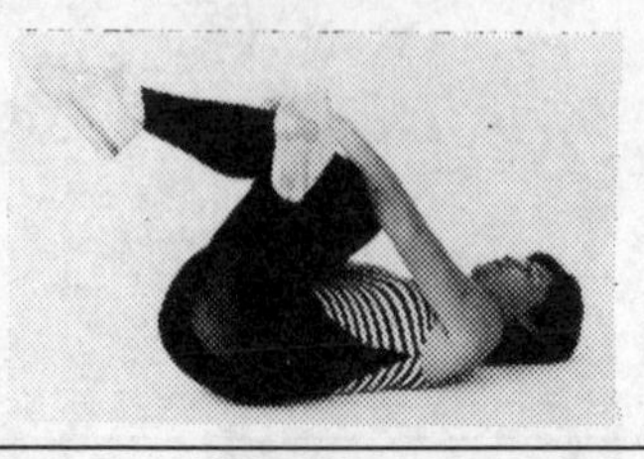

Cross your legs as shown. Pull your knees towards your chest. This will stretch your gluteals and lower back. Hold the stretch 8-10 seconds then reverse your leg cross. Repeat.

DANGER

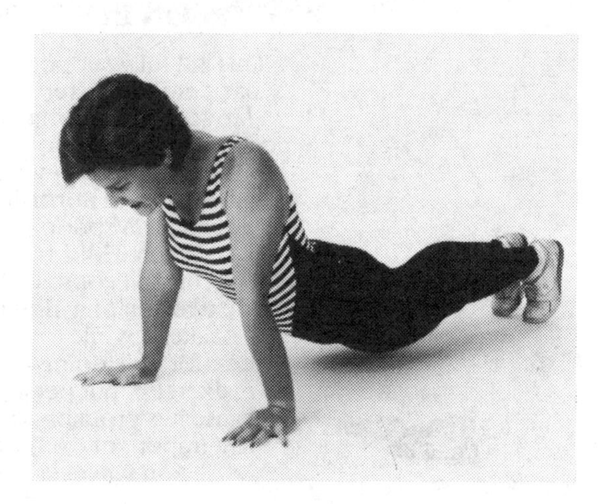

SAGGING PUSH-UPS

The push-up is designed to strengthen and tone your upper-body. Especially your chest and triceps.

The most common problem when executing this exercise is sagging of the hips. This not only forces the body weight onto your upper-legs, therefore, reducing the workload for your upper-body, it also causes extension compression in your lower spine.

Again, poor execution of a potentially safe exercise will reduce the desired effect, and make injury a real possibility.

If you feel your body sagging, revert back to a lower intensity exercise until your strength is sufficient to progress to the full body position.

Sagging in stonger people often occurs when too many repetitions are attempted in one set.

Some people have very flexible elbow joints, but try to avoid locking your elbows at the top of the push-ups. Joint locking may occur as you tire. Reduce your number of repetitions if this is the case.

DANGER RATING: Very High

SAFE ALTERNATIVES

HALF PUSH-UP

This is the starting point for every person who wants to begin to build upper-body strength. You will reduce the intensity of this push-up by putting your weight back over your knees.

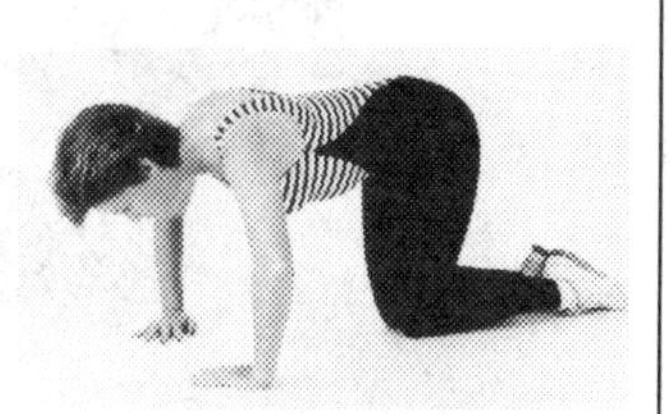

THREE-QUARTER PUSH-UP

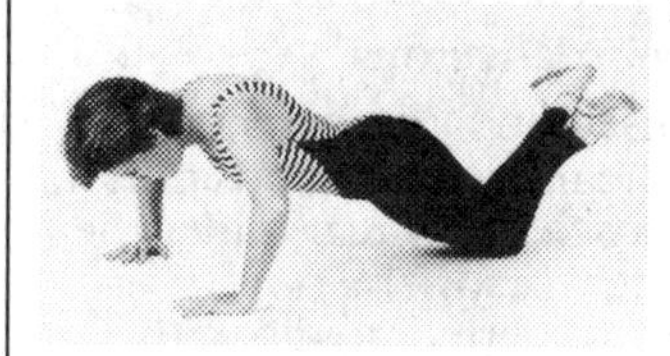

Your workload is increased by placing more upper-body weight over your arms. Lifting the feet increases the workload a little more.

FULL PUSH-UP

The full body press sould be your goal. A daily schedule of this exercise will develop good upper-body and arm strength. But remember to progress slowly from the lower intensity work.

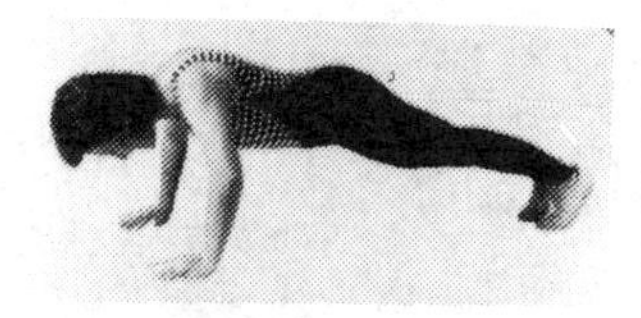

CHAIR PUSH-UP

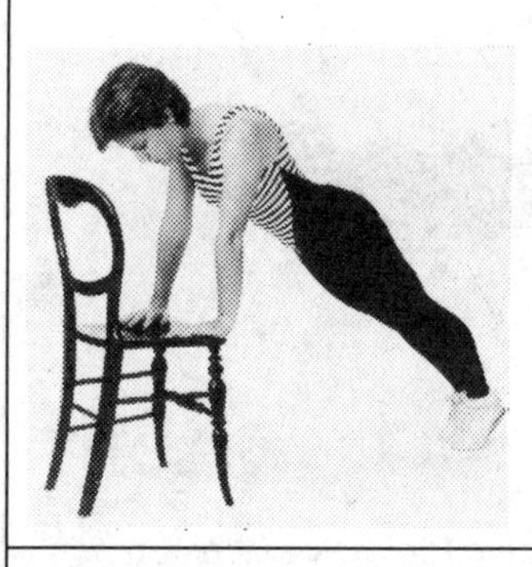

If you have knee trouble, use a chair, bench, sofa or wall to reduce the workload, and reduce the stress on your knees. Using the wall will still give you a good toning effect if you do the exercise regularly and include 20-30 repetitions in each set.

RELAX & STRETCH

It is desirable to stretch the upper back, chest and arm muscles after push-ups. Assume the position shown and stretch your arms along the floor. People with knee problems should use a wall.

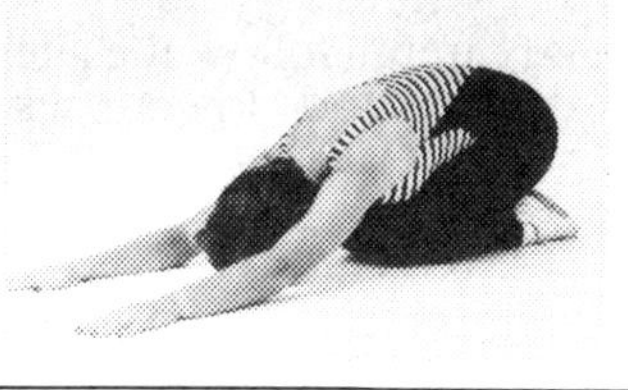

DANGER

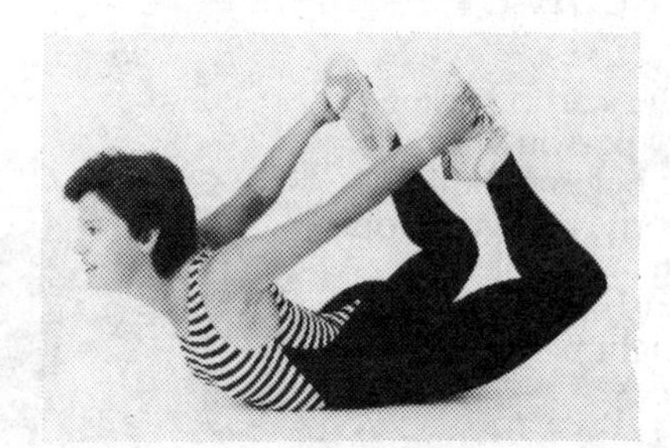

BANANA BENDS

You may also remember this exercise being completed with arms and legs raised off the ground but without the hands holding the ankles.

Both positions are potentially dangerous.

The holding position because you hyperextend and compress your spine, and the non-holding position because your lower back muscles may tear under the weight of your legs and upper-torso. The non-holding position also produces vertebral, disc and nerve compression.

DANGER RATING: Very High

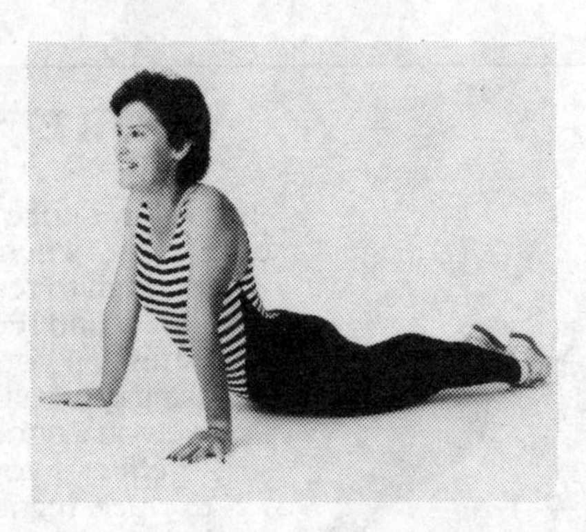

THE COBRA

The cobra is a safer alternative for back extension exercises, which are necessary to help maintain lower back mobility.

The only danger in the cobra occurs when you force the extension too far and begin to create excessive compression forces on your discs, vertebrae and emerging nerve supply. Vertebral fractures and dislocation can occur.

Be careful, follow the alternatives and you will develop good lower-back strength, and mobility, without risk.

DANGER RATING: High

SAFE ALTERNATIVES

COBRA ON ELBOWS

This is a fully supported back mobility exercise. Move to a comfortable position and hold. Do not force the arch in your back. You will normally also feel an abdominal stretch. Hold 10-20 seconds. People with poor extension may find it takes a while to feel comfortable doing this exercise, but persist, because it is probably the most important exercise you will ever do.

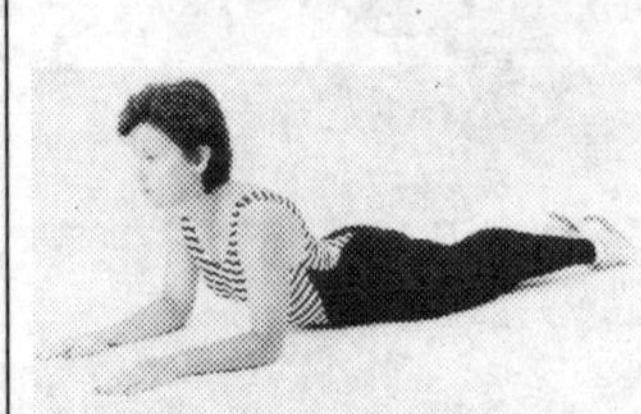

LEG LIFT

A fully supported strengthening exercise for your lower back. Lift one leg at a time. Raise and lower in one slow but continuous movement. Repeat 6 to 8 times with each leg, rest, and repeat again. This exercise also works the gluteals.

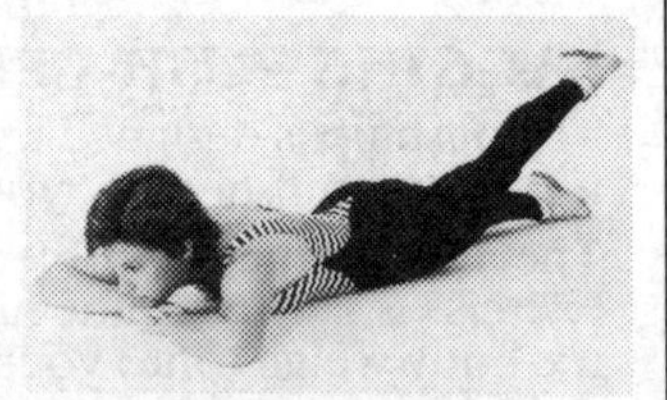

ARM AND LEG LIFT

This increases the intensity of your workload, and also includes strengthening for your upper back. Always work your opposite arm and leg and move slowly and continuously, as with the single leg lift.

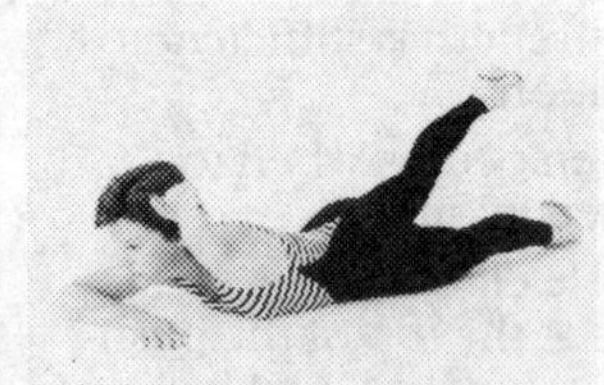

CAT CURL

Curl your back as shown. You should feel a stretch in your upper back and shoulders. Hold 8-10 seconds then relax. Do not sag your stomach and back when relaxing.

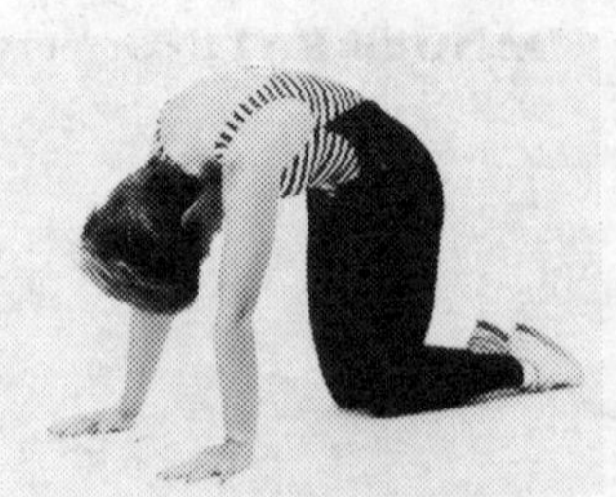

BACK TWIST

Hold this position 10-20 seconds and repeat 3 times each side. Do not force yourself past the point of a pleasant stretch. Good for lower back mobility and gluteal stretch.

DANGER

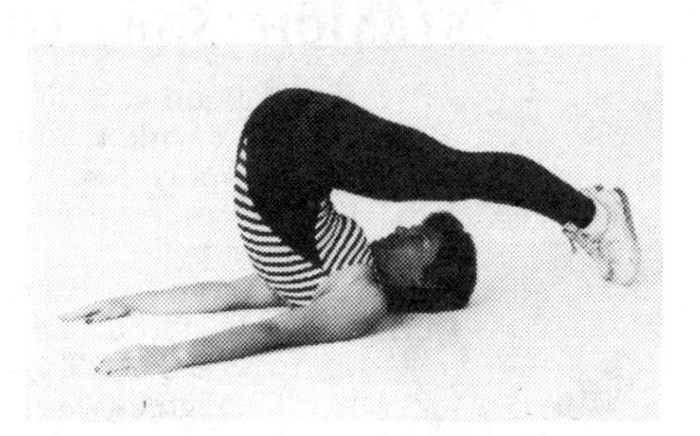

PLOW — CERVICAL FLEXION WITH WEIGHT

Resting heavy bodyweight on your neck is obviously not a very good idea.

The cervical region of your neck is very delicate and compression damage to your discs, vertebrae, or nerves, can occur.

Overstretching the surrounding ligaments may cause vertebral movement and produce pressure on the nerve supply to your arms, upper-torso, neck and head.

Referred arm pain and headaches may result.

DANGER RATING: Extreme

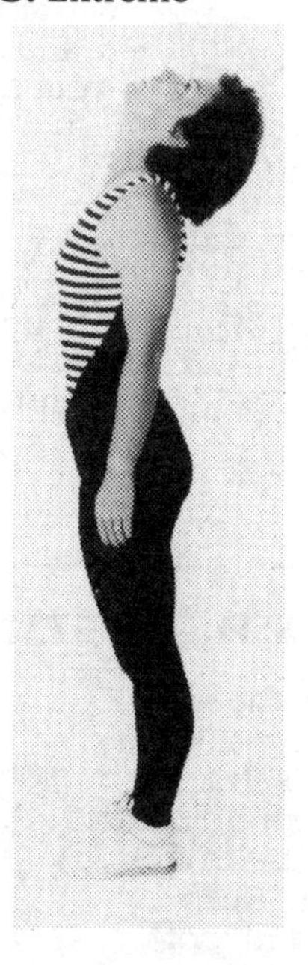

CERVICAL HYPEREXTENSION

Anyone who has suffered whiplash injuries in a car accident will tell you of the chronic pain and discomfort that occurs from cervical spine damage.

Hyperextension and hyperflexion exercises are extremely dangerous and should not be included in your exercise programme, unless prescribed by a qualified medical professional for mobility or strengthening purposes.

Muscle tension in the neck and upper back is best relieved by massage, or by using the alternative exercises opposite.

DANGER RATING: Extreme

SAFE ALTERNATIVES

HEAD FORWARD

Lower your head forward and fix your eyes approximately two metres in front of your feet. This will stretch the muscles in your upper back and neck. Do not force your head down.

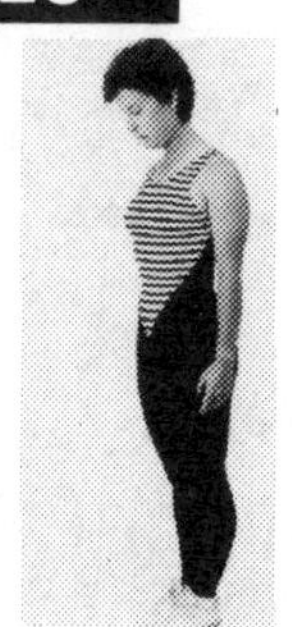

SIDE NECK STRENGTH

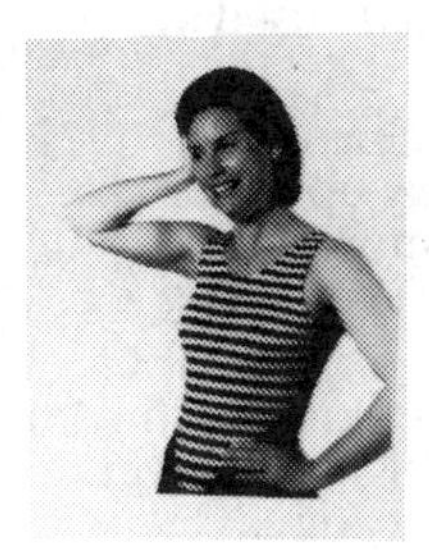

Force your head against your hand and hold for 5 seconds. Repeat 3 times on both sides. Your hand only offers resistance, it does not force your head back. This is an isometric strengthening exercise and should not be done by people with high blood pressure.

FORWARD NECK STRENGTH

This is a strengthening exercise for sterno-mastoid and other muscles in the side and front of your neck. Perform the same as the previous exercise. Do not force your head back, and stop immediately if you feel any discomfort.

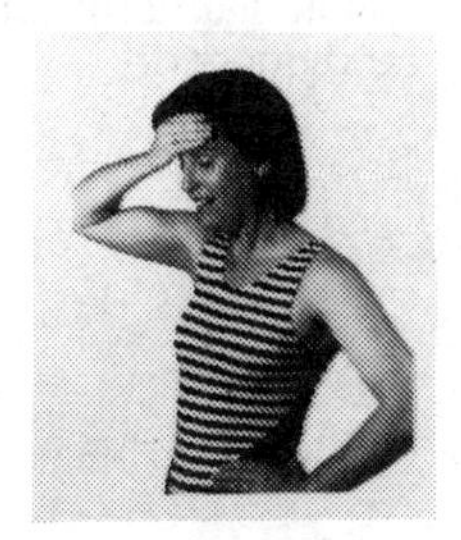

EAR TO SHOULDER

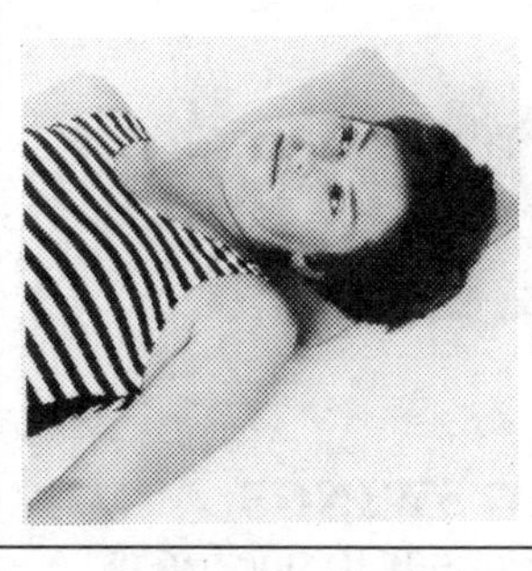

Relax your upper back, chest and neck muscles. Place your head gently to one side to stretch the opposite side muscles. Do not force this position. Keep your head on the pillow. This exercise will improve cervical mobility and relieve spinal compression in this region.

HEAD ROLLS

Keep the weight of your head well supported on a small pillow. Look slowly from side to side and roll your head gently across the pillow. This will assist you to increase your cervical spine mobility. Move your head very slowly and do not force your neck to turn past the point of pleasant comfort.

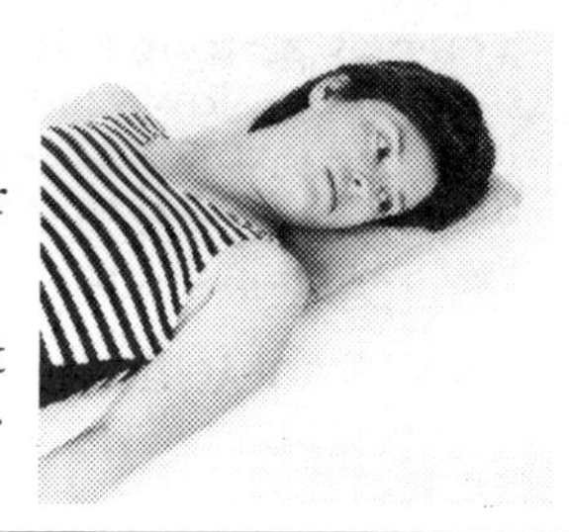

DANGER

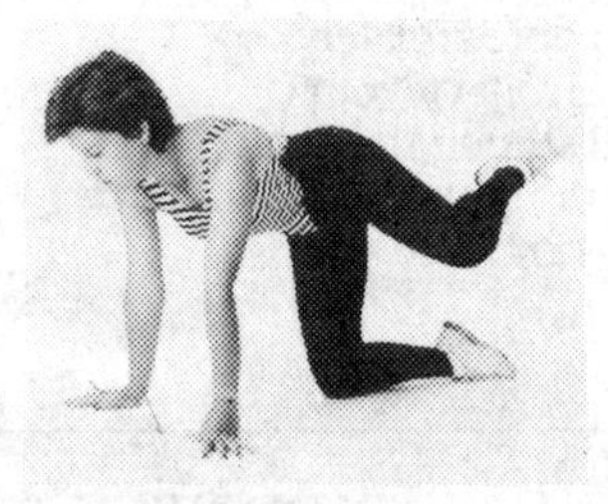

RAPID SIDE LEG RAISES

Another hip-toning exercise commonly used in aerobic exercise classes.

In too many classes, however, participants are encouraged to throw their leg rapidly upwards — twisting the spine and putting enormous strain on the muscles and ligaments of the supporting leg and hip.

This exercise should always be done slowly and with control. **DO NOT** raise the leg too high and never do more than 8-10 repetitions at any one time.

DANGER RATING: The very small hip rotating muscles are in extreme danger during "rapid side leg raises". The stabilising hip ligaments are also in extreme danger, while your lower back muscles, spinal ligaments and lumbar nerves may easily be damaged.

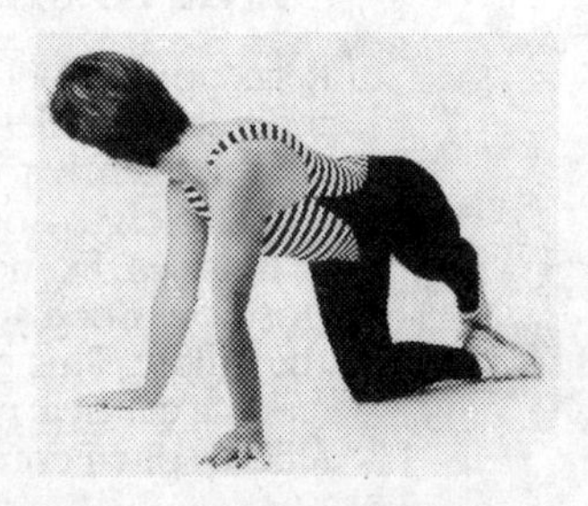

RAPID STRAIGHT LEG SWINGS

Rapidly swinging your leg from side to side forces the spine to twist and bend violently. The potential damage to nerves, ligaments, discs, vertebrae and back muscles makes this a very poor quality and dangerous exercise.

You may perform this exercise safely if you move the leg very slowly and in a very controlled manner. It should help tone your hips, buttocks and inside thigh muscles if done correctly.

Fast swinging of the leg is **DEFINITELY OUT.**

DANGER RATING: Extreme.

SAFE ALTERNATIVES

STRAIGHT SIDE-LEG LIFT

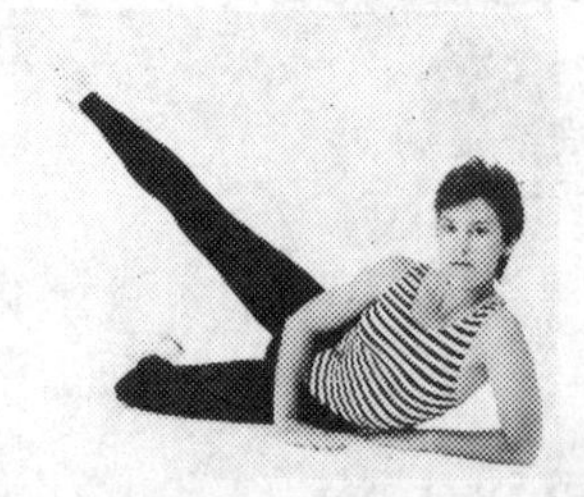

Bend your floor leg to widen your base of support. Keep your hip, knee and foot of the lifting leg in line. Raise and lower your leg in a slow and controlled manner. **DO NOT** go past 45 degrees. Great for the abductor muscles — your hips and bottom.

BENT SIDE-LEG LIFT

This is an alternative to "side-leg raises" on your knees. It is low intensity work and removes the stress on your supporting hip. Perform the same as the straight side-leg lift.

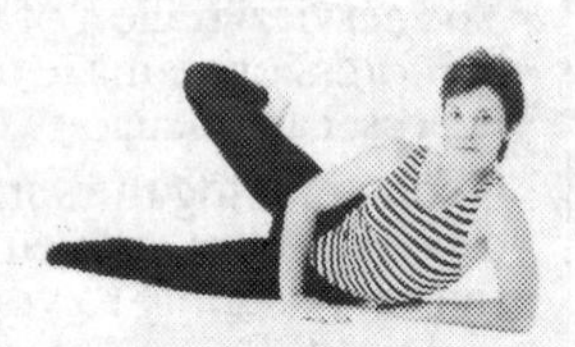

KNEE AND TOE TAP

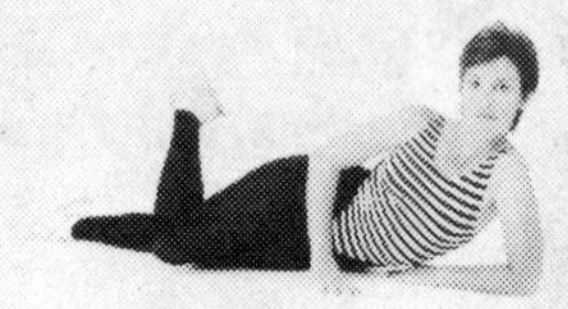

Move to tap your knee and toe on either side of your supporting leg. Keep your movements slow and controlled. Rest comfortably on your elbow and **DO NOT** push up too high. This will prevent excessive side flexion of your spine. The controlled elbow rest will give you extra spine mobility work.

STANDING SIDE-LEG LIFT

This is probably the safest and most effective side-leg lift. Your spine is straight, your body supported and the abductor muscles are isolated to work. Keep your hip, knee and foot aligned. Raise and lower your leg with control.

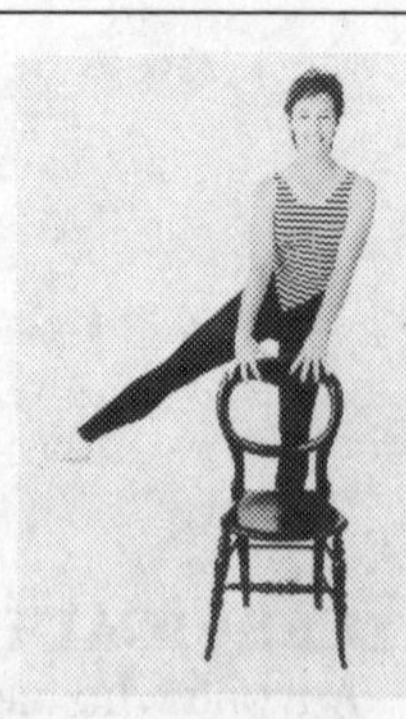

SPINAL ROTATIONS

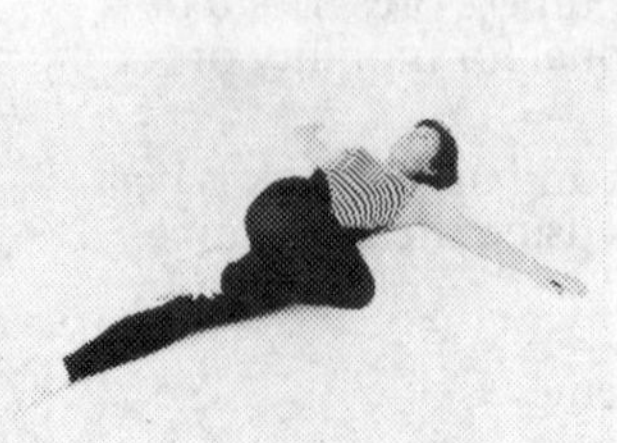

Bend one leg up and roll over your straight leg. **DO NOT** force this position. Move only to a point of pleasant stretch. Good for your gluteals and lower back mobility. Hold this position for 10-20 seconds.

DANGER

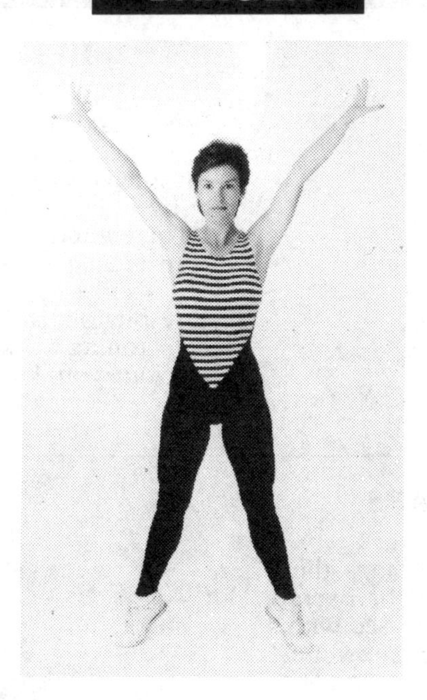

STAR JUMPS

You may know these as astride jumps or jumping jacks.

Star jumps are a commonly used but very dangerous exercise.

As a two-foot bouncing exercise, star jumps produce excessive vertical forces which create undue stress on your ankle, knee, hip and vertebral joints.

Recent research has shown that these forces are 5 to 6 times the vertical forces experienced during walking, and 2 to 3 times the forces felt during jogging.

The exact force difference does not matter. The fact remains that continual two-foot bouncing will result in joint damage or "the dreaded" shin splints.

There is also some research suggesting that star jumps cause minor nerve dysfunctioning.

Women who suffer from **STRESS INCONTINENCE** are doubly disadvantaged.

The internal abdominal forces produced during star jumps place the bladder under enormous pressure, and women who have weak pelvic floor muscles suffer urine leakage with such pressure.

PELVIC FLOOR EXERCISES are a must. It is recommended that all females complete at least 50 quality pelvic floor contractions every day.

Stopping your urine mid-flow is a test of pelvic floor strength.

Star jumps should be eliminated from your exercise programme.

DANGER RATING: Extreme

SAFE ALTERNATIVES

SKIPPING

Skipping from foot to foot reduces significantly the impact stress. Use a rope where possible and move around to reduce the vertical forces on your legs and spine. A moderate intensity cardio-respiratory exercise. **DO NOT** lock your knees.

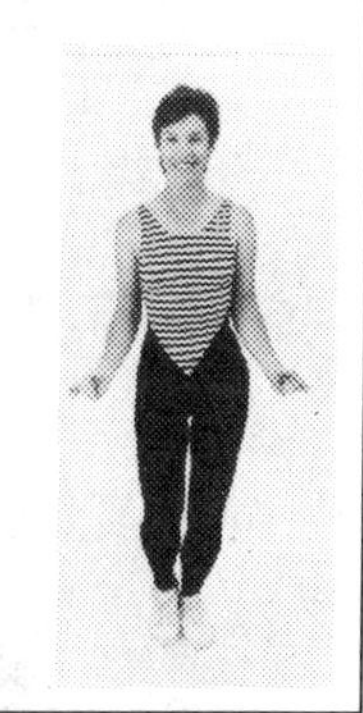

STEP-TOUCH

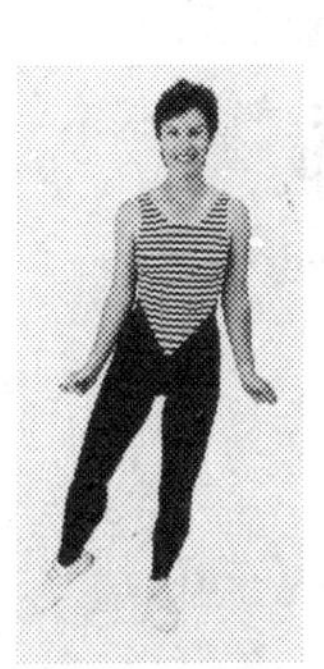

Stepping exercises offer excellent low impact activities. You may increase your work intensity by higher leg lifts or wider steps. Good horizontal moves for confined spaces where full walking steps are not possible.

BOX STEP

Step right, cross left, step back right and step side left. Another low impact dance step. Often used in aerobic dance classes. Again, the intensity may be increased by running.

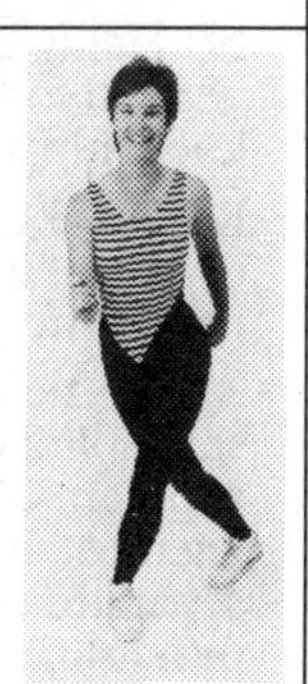

WALKING

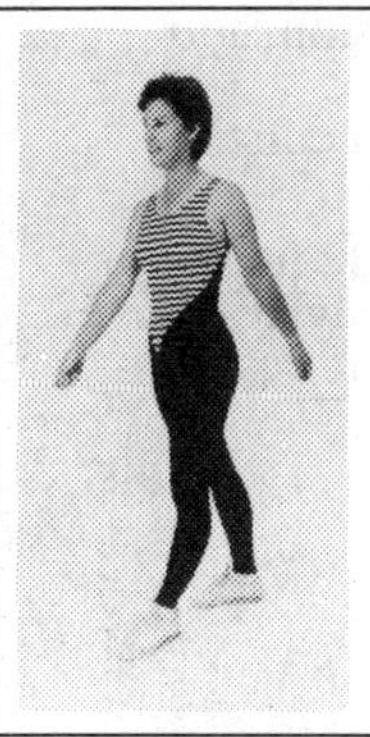

This is probably the safest form of leg endurance and cardiovascular exercise. Highly recommended. Walk briskly for 20-30 minutes every second day for an effective fitness programme.

JAZZ WALKING

There are many jazz dance steps used in aerobic classes. All offer a variety of horizontal movements with greater safety and effectiveness than jumping up and down on the spot.

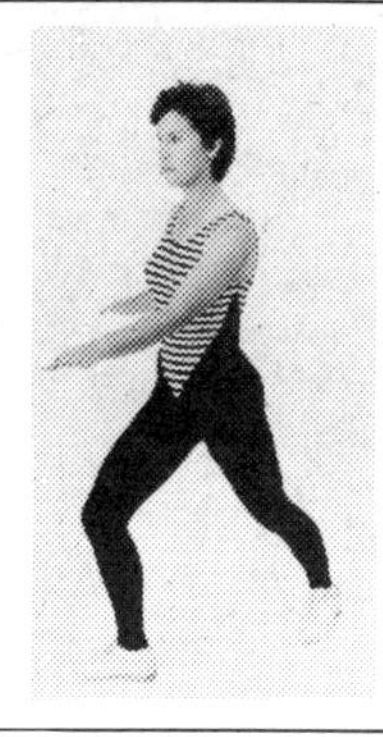

DANGER

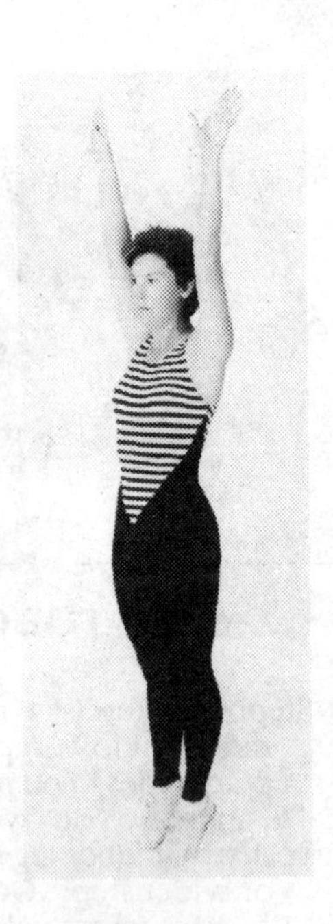
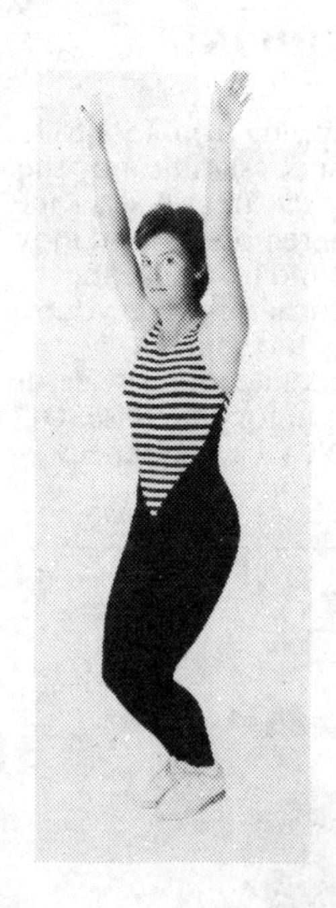

DOUBLE TOE BOUNCING

This exercise has all the inherent problems, and possible dangers, of star jumps.

Bouncing up and down on the spot creates large vertical forces which must be absorbed by the ankle, knee, hip and intervertebral joints.

Recent U.S. studies have shown that over 85 percent of instructors, who repetitively bounce on the spot, have suffered some form of injury.

Again, the most common injury is shin soreness or shin splints. This may be caused by a variety of problems, including over-development of the lower-leg musculature (compartment syndrome), separation of tendons from other tendons or bone, or hairline fractures of the tibia or fibula.

Intervertebral discs also suffer compression, and "double toe bouncing" quickens the disc degeneration process which normally occurs with age.

DO NOT perform any exercises which require you to two foot bounce on the spot. Try to always move horizontally or perform low impact exercises.

DANGER RATING: Extreme

SAFE ALTERNATIVES

HEEL TAPS

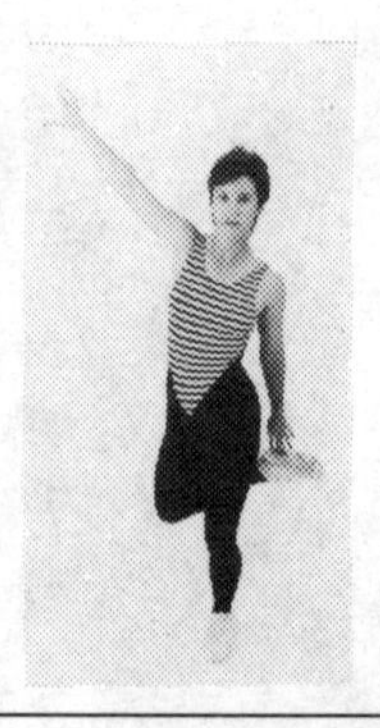

Step and tap your heel behind your leg. Increase the intensity of this work by adding a small hop. This exercise combines arm and leg movements, and is good cardio-respiratory and muscle toning work. Avoid locking your knee joint.

CALF TAPS

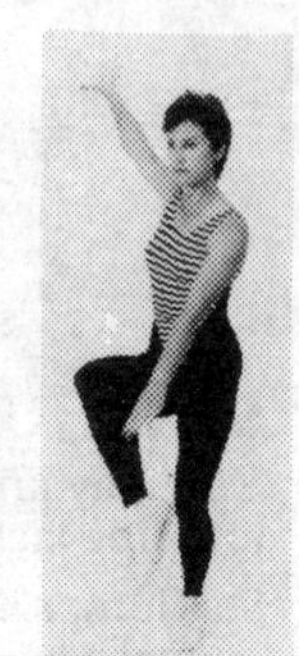

As with heel taps, the intensity of this exercise can be increased with a hop. In both exercises you should keep your back straight and your abdominal muscles pulled tightly in to avoid any chance of injury.

STEP KICK

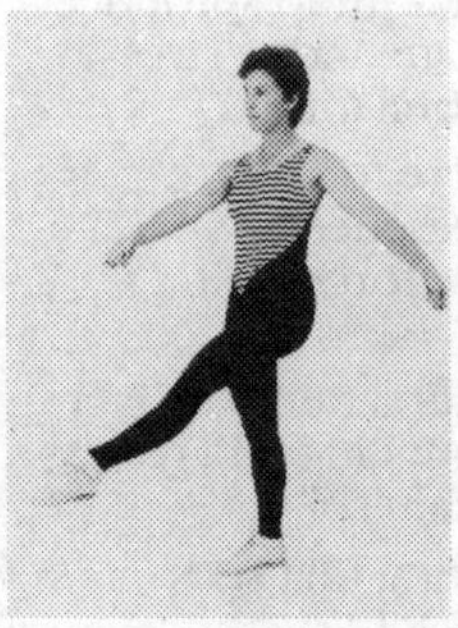

Stepping and walking exercises are probably the safest form of exercise. Add a kick for variety and increased intensity. Make sure your kick is controlled.

GRAPE-VINE STEP

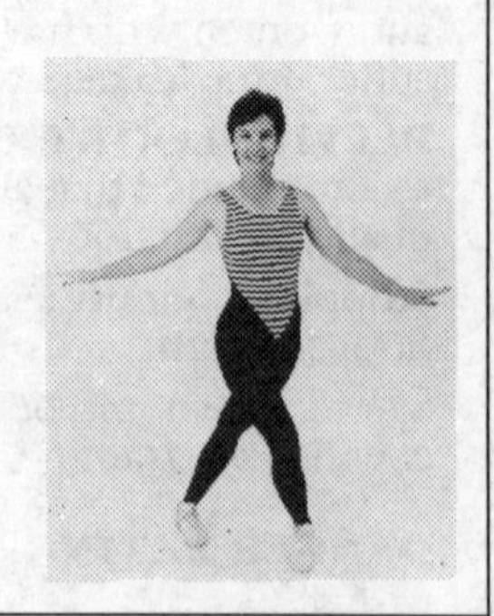

Moving sideways placing your trailing leg firstly in-front and then behind the leading leg. There are many traditional or contemporary dance steps that may be used in your exercise programme. Avoid moving and twisting too quickly or knee injury may occur.

STEP-BALL CHANGE

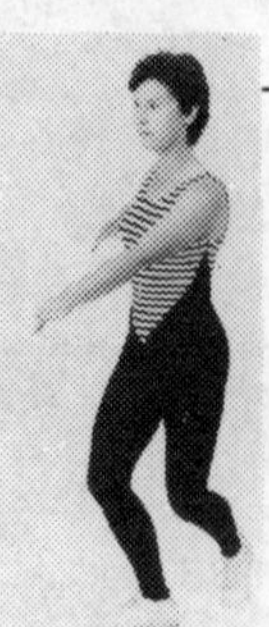

A common jazz step with a small skip in between each step. Safe, effective and great when working in small groups.

DANGER

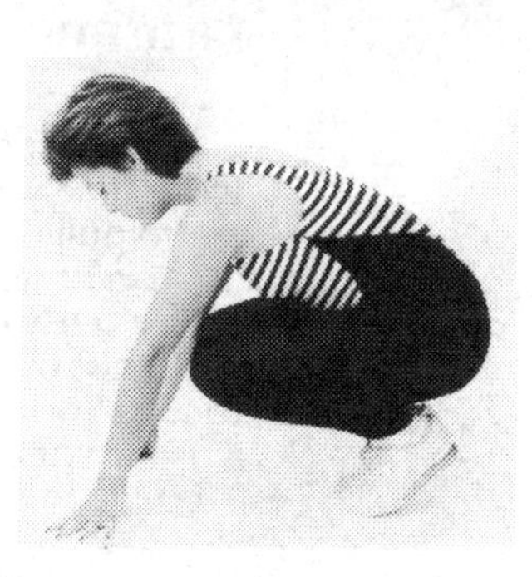

BURPEES
This is a muscular endurance cum cardiovascular activity which is dreaded by even the toughest and strongest of football players.

It is very tiring, and the execution of the double leg kick-out leaves most people in a "sagging push-up" position.

This is a definite "no-no" for the unconditioned, and one to watch for the more advanced.

Ballistic sagging in the lower back region can be extremely damaging, as can the constant two foot bouncing when you jump upright.

DANGER RATING: Very High

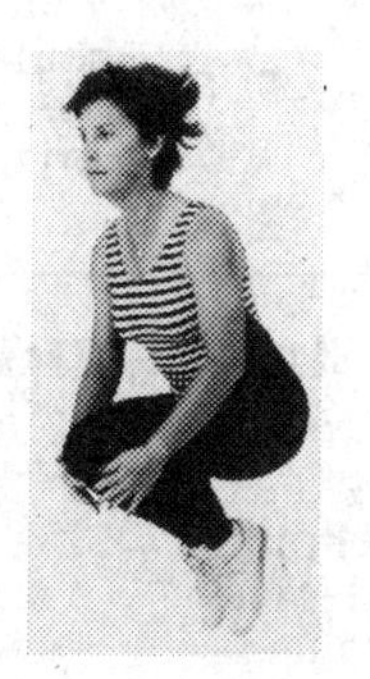

TUCK JUMPS
Some people add the tuck jump to increase their work-load.

This exercise, however, produces even greater vertical forces than double-toe bouncing or star jumps. Compression damage to your spine is very likely.

Don't risk the injury. Go for a nice brisk walk or swim. Forget these exercises completely.

DANGER RATING: Very High

SAFE ALTERNATIVES

CHEST STRETCH

Use a chair, wall or partner. Turn until you feel a pleasant stretch in your chest. A must after push-ups, Russians or any upper-body work.

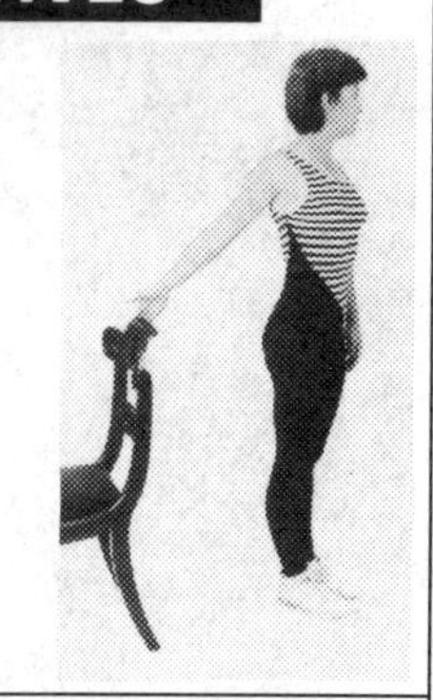

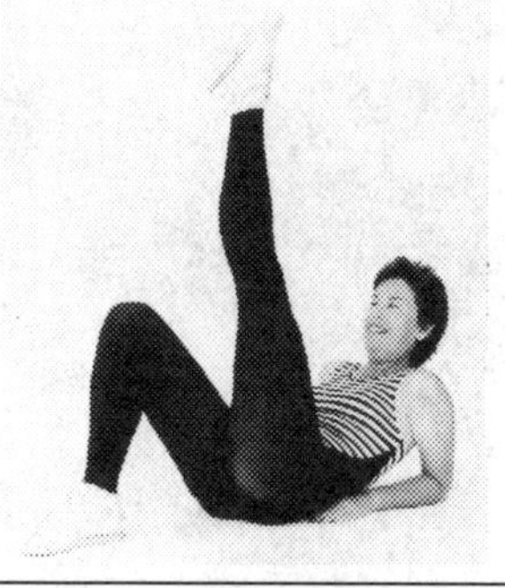

RUSSIANS FLOOR

This exercise requires you to kick your legs up and down alternately. Resting on your elbows reduces stress on your back and wrists. **NEVER** CYCLE YOUR LEGS.

RUSSIANS HIGH

An advanced exercise with increased workload. If you have blood pressure or wrist problems revert back to "Russians floor". Keep your head up and your back straight.

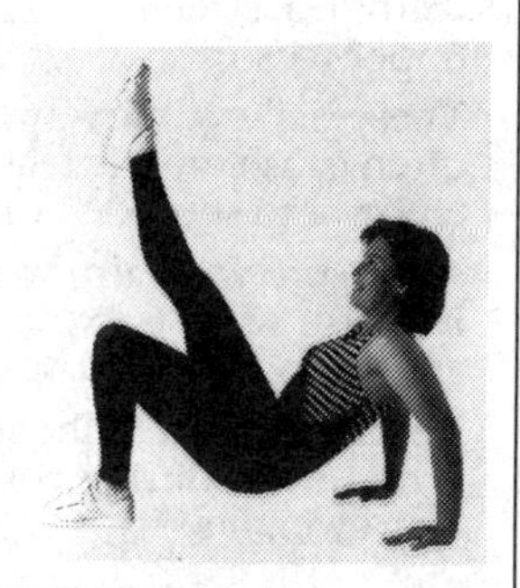

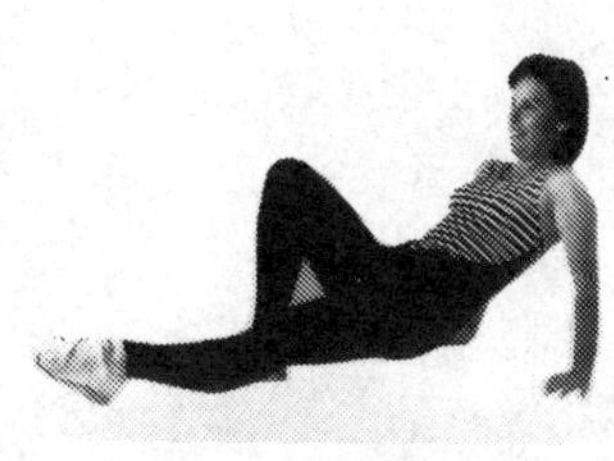

DIP AND KICK

You can increase the intensity of your exercise by working your arms and legs simultaneously. Step your legs alternately while you dip with your arms.

FLOOR TOUCHES

The closest there is to a burpee without all the jarring. Walk forward 4 steps, bend and touch the ground as shown. Keep your back straight and step back to the upright position. Repeat.

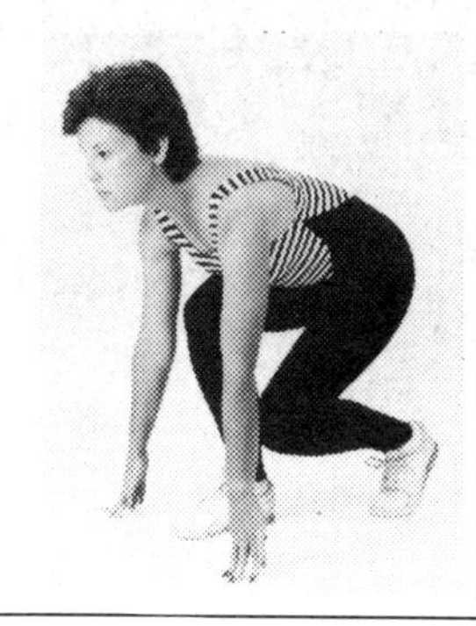

DANGER

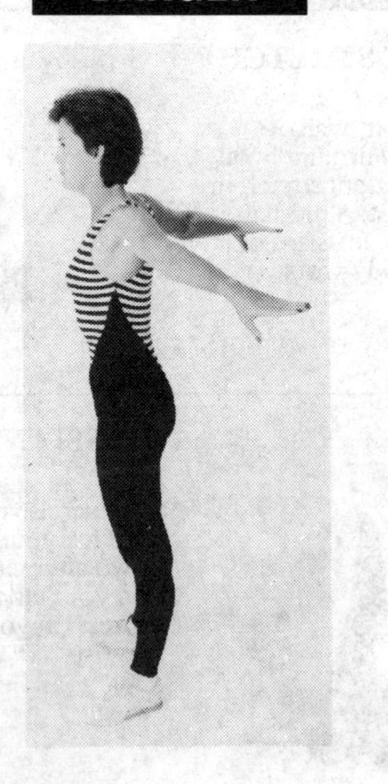

FAST ARM FLINGS

Many people use arm flinging exercises to help warm-up, stretch or tone muscles in the arms and upper-torso.

These ballistic movements are very dangerous. They often cause muscle tears, and ligament damage in elbow and shoulder joints.

Make sure your arm work is controlled at all times. Fast arm work is extremely dangerous for elderly and unconditioned people.

Toning and strengthening of muscles in this region is best done during your floorwork, or with light hand weights.

DANGER RATING: High

SAFE ALTERNATIVES

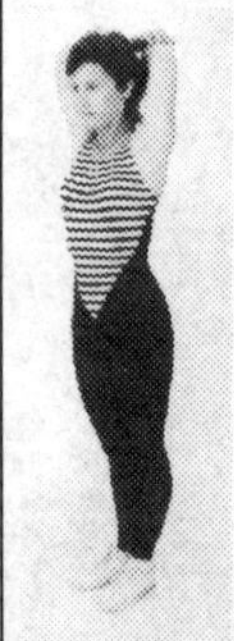

TRICEPS STRETCH

A must after any arm work. Use your free hand to pull the stretch to a point where you feel pleasantly comfortable. Do not over stretch the triceps. Hold each stretch for 8-10 seconds.

SHOULDER STRETCH

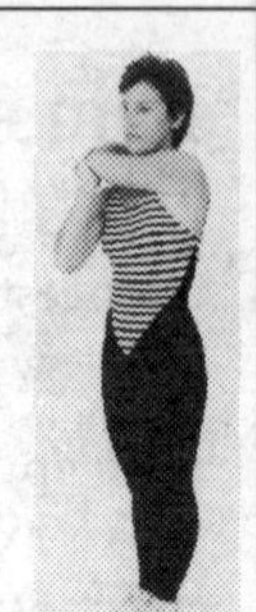

Put your arm across your chest and hold with your support arm. Move to a pleasant stretch and hold. Add a body twist if you wish to include muscles in the upper back.

CURLS WITH SMALL WEIGHTS

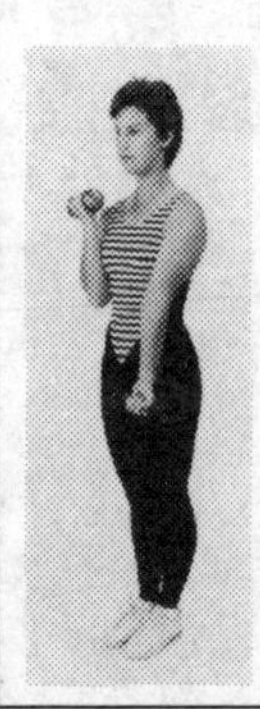

Use cans of food, books or small weights of any description. Elastic bands offer good resistance but are dangerous if they break during the exercise. The weight will increase your work intensity and help you slow down the movement. This is a bicep curl using alternate arms.

FLYS WITH SMALL WEIGHTS

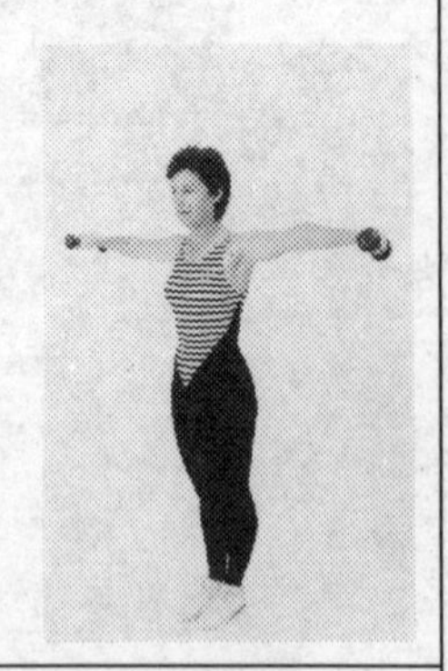

This exercise works mainly on your deltoid muscles. Raise and lower from the side of your body, 90 degrees to the horizontal. Repetitions should be slow and continuous. A good strengthening exercise even without the hand weights.

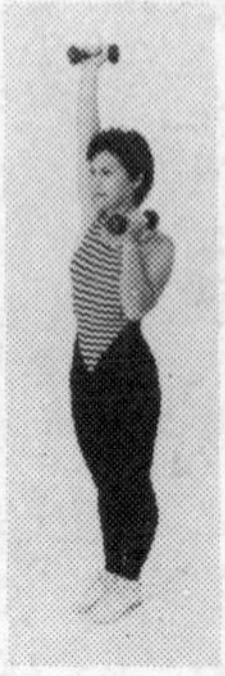

OVERHEAD PRESS

Again, movements should be well controlled. Press above the head with alternate arms. Keep your back straight and your abdominals contracted. Attention to posture and technique is important in all exercising.

DANGER

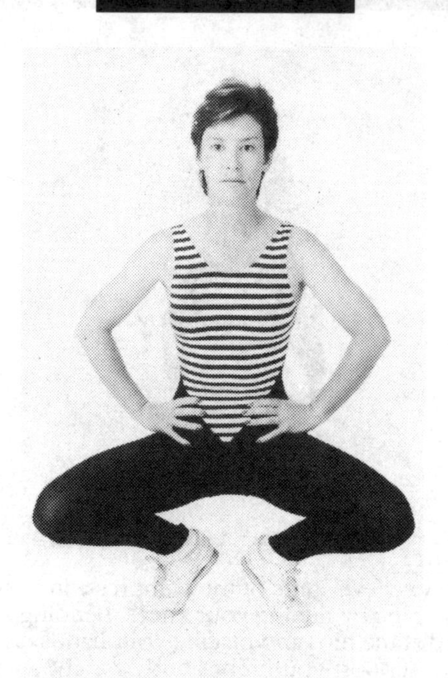

DEEP KNEE BENDS

You will remember that bending at the knees is essential to safe lifting techniques.

But you will also remember that even when lifting, your knees should not bend more than 90 degrees.

Once you pass through the 90 degree limit, you will be performing a deep knee bend.

At this point, the forces exerted on your knee caps and surrounding ligaments, muscles and tendons are greatly multiplied.

These forces may cause injury to any of the structures around the knees, including the cartilage.

This exercise is completely unnecessary for general fitness.

You will even notice that weight lifters often heavily bandage their knees to help support the surrounding structures and minimize the potential for injury.

DANGER RATING: Very High

SAFE ALTERNATIVES

QUARTER SQUATS

A simple, low intensity, no-impact exercise for all fitness levels. Controlled and varied arm coordination work will help increase the intensity of this exercise.

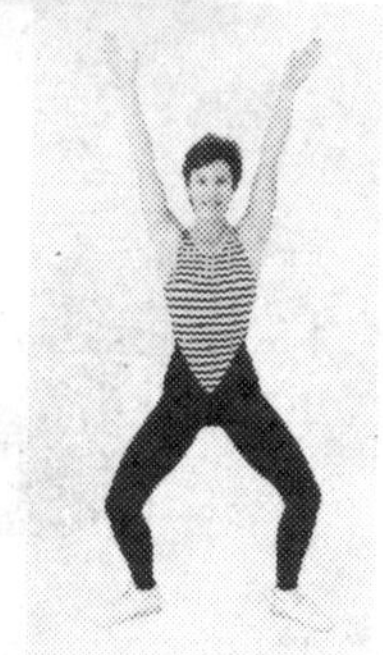

KNEELING — STEP UP & DOWN

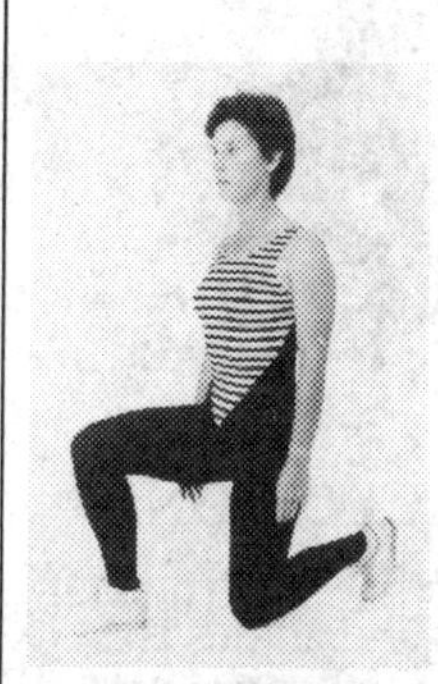

This is a more intense exercise which requires good balance. Step forward, bend both knees as shown. Rest on one knee while bringing your other leg to the kneeling position. Step back up with your first kneeling leg until you are standing upright. Repeat. Avoid if you have any knee problems.

FOOT TO CHAIR

A low to moderate intensity exercise. Step to just touch the edge of the chair. Increase the intensity by using a higher chair. Keep your back straight and tummy flat.

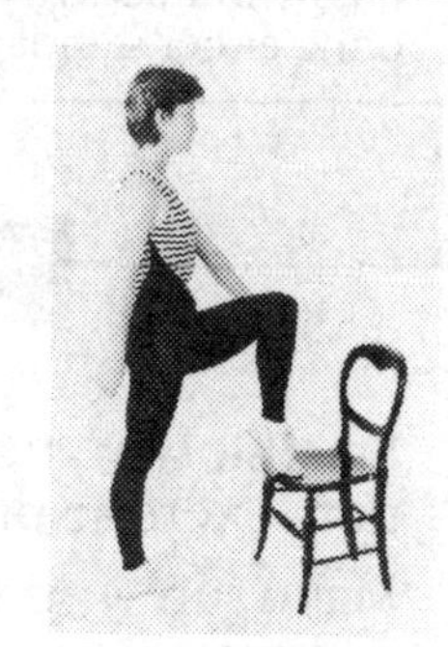

LUNGE

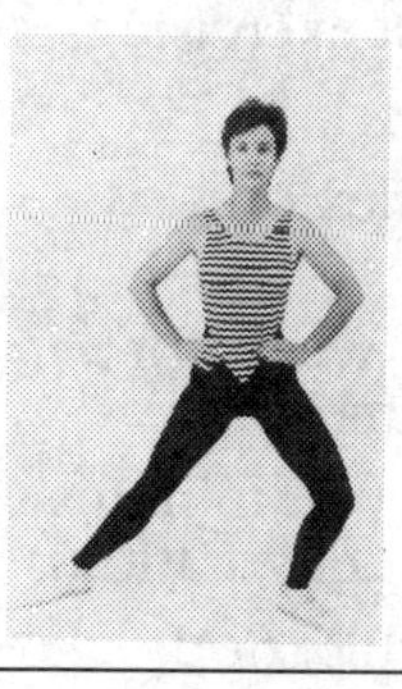

Controlled side lunges are a very good alternative to deep squats. Move slowly from side to side keeping your feet pointing in the direction of your knee flexion. All the above exercises increase quadricep strength.

QUADRICEPS STRETCH

A must at the end of any thigh work. You will attain your best stretch with your body fully supported in the lying position.

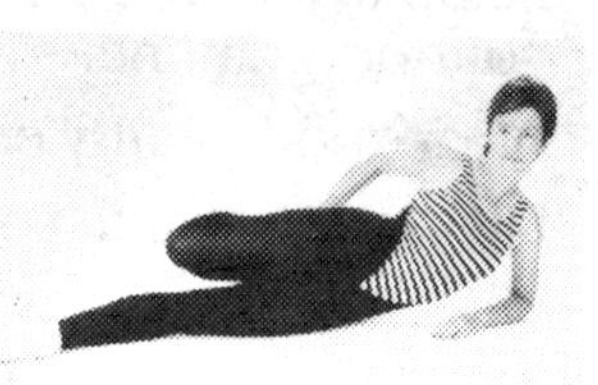

ALSO AVOID

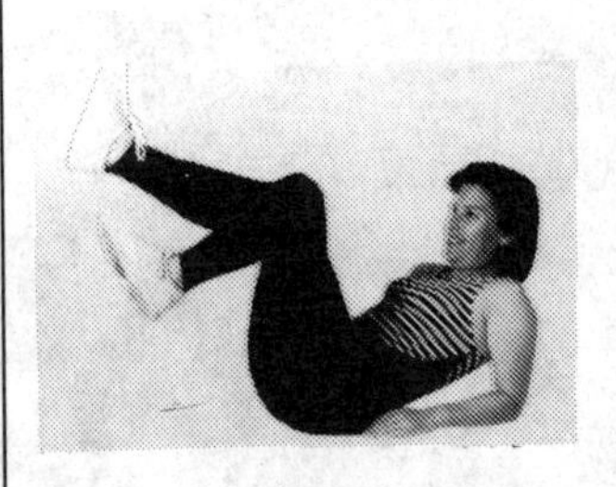

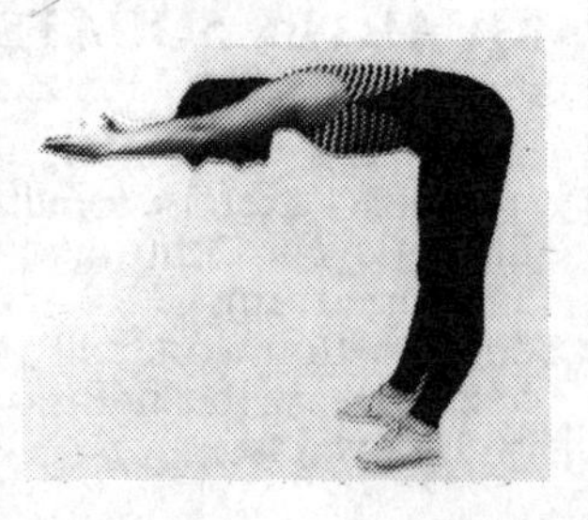

CYCLING **FLAT BACK BEND**

Both these exercises also put excessive strain on your spine and have minimal fitness benefits.

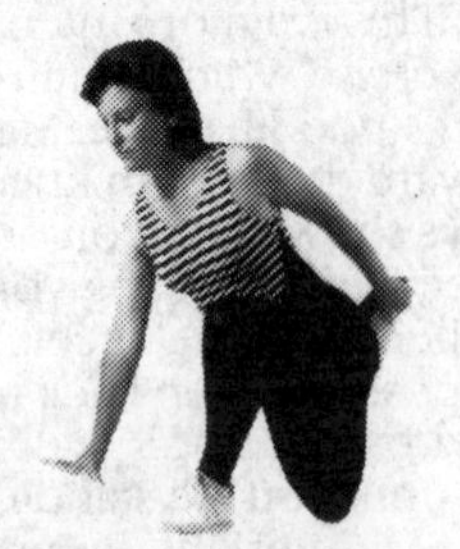

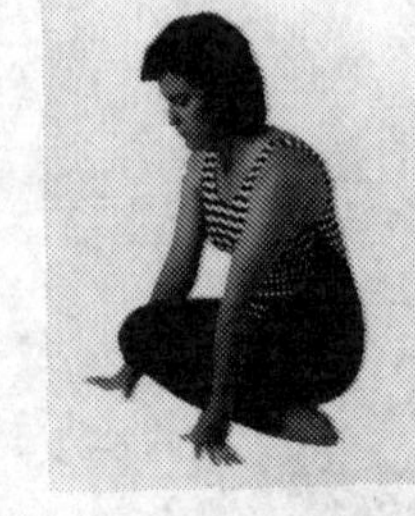

STRETCH ON KNEES **STRETCH ON ANKLES**

Putting extra pressure on your knees and ankles is totally unnecessary. All lower limb stretches are best done either standing upright or lying down.

SPINAL COMPRESSION RELIEF

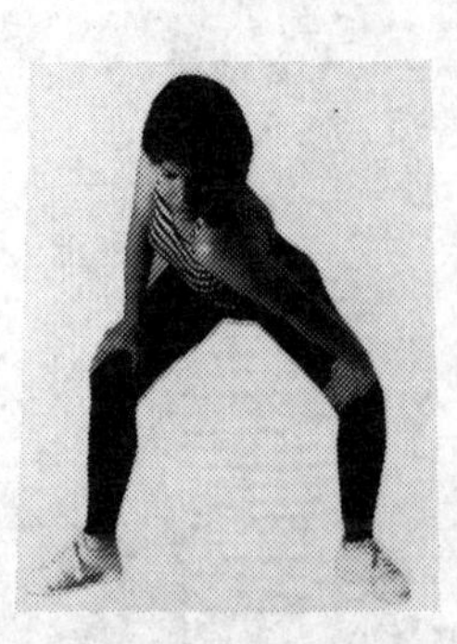

You may relieve some of the compression in your lumbar spine by flexing your knees, bending forward at the hips and placing your hands on your knees to support your upper-body weight.

Once in this position you should slowly twist and dip your shoulders.

You will feel some separation and relief in the lumbar vertebrae, and pleasant stretching of muscles in your lower back.

Compression relief work is essential in all exercise programmes.

ALWAYS

Start slowly and progress gradually with any new exercise programme.

Make sure you warm up properly before every workout.

Static stretch all major muscle groups before any fast, full range of movement exercising.

Protect your spine and lower back.

Do a balance of extension and flexion exercises for spinal mobility.

Exercise regularly 3-5 times per week, for a minimum of 20 minutes each time.

Drink a glass of cold water every 20 minutes of vigorous exercise to prevent dehydration.

Include a cool-down and stretch period after vigorous activity.

Include cardiovascular, muscle toning, flexibility and spinal mobility work in your programme.

Wear good quality exercise shoes.

Eat a low fat, high complex carbohydrate diet.

Vary your activities to beat boredom.

NEVER

Start an exercise programme without answering **"THE TEST"** on page 4.

Stretch your muscles beyond the point of pleasant comfort.

Exercise vigorously in very humid or very hot climatic conditions.

Hold your breath during physical activity.

Hyperventilate during exercise or at rest.

Work through pain.

Exercise through illness or injury.

Stand still immediately after vigorous physical activity.

Exercise on hard concrete surfaces.

Exercise in crowded and poorly ventilated rooms.

Perform any dangerous exercise.

Sacrifice quality for quantity. Never exercise through fatigue.

LOWER LIMB CARE

LOWER LIMBS AND FEET

It is important to always take good care of your feet and legs. They are your most prominent means of exercising, and any injury will limit your fitness programme.

You may have bowed legs, or knocked knees, or one leg shorter than the other. Or you may, as many women find, have a wide pelvis which causes the joint angle at your knee to produce excessive rubbing under the knee cap. This condition is known as Chondromalacia.

Be aware that any of these leg problems may promote muscle, tendon, ligament or cartilage injuries.

Your legs may also either pronate or supinate excessively when running, skipping or brisk walking.

Excessive rolling in (pronation), or rolling out (supination) at the ankle will eventually cause leg injury.

All the above conditions, plus others, normally require assessment by a Podiatrist, or Medical Practitioner, before a successful corrective programme can be developed.

In many instances, altering the cushioning of your shoes by specially made orthotics is all that is needed.

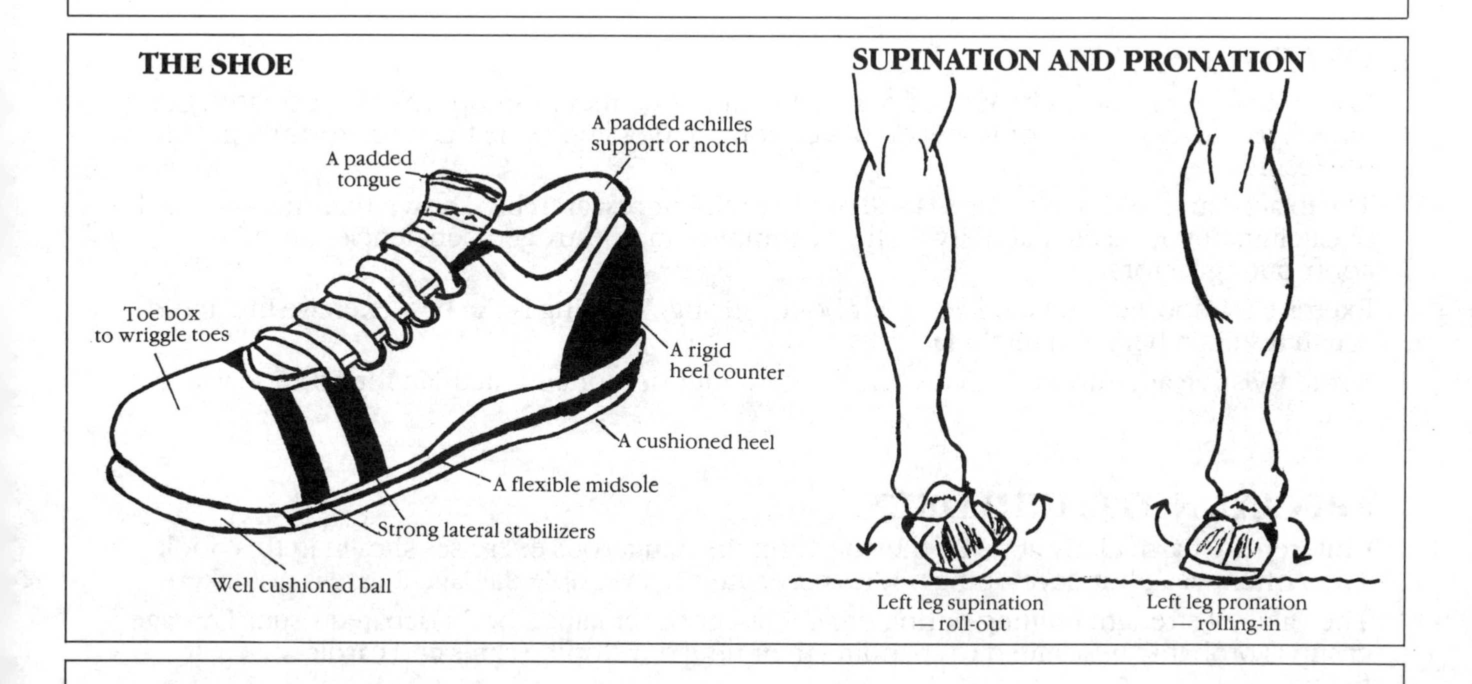

SELECTING AN EXERCISE SHOE

When selecting your exercise shoe, you need to consider your foot type, the nature of your activity, and the surface on which you are going to work.

A shoe fits properly if you are able to wriggle your toes, but still feel firm support and do not slide back and forward inside the shoe.

The better exercise shoes have a soft raised heel wedge, padded tongue, a flexible and shock resistant midsole, a firm heel counter, good lateral stabilizers and appropriate arch support.

Flared soles are good for running activities while the more rounded soles are better for the side to side movements normally associated with aerobic classess.

Where possible, avoid shoes with curved soles unless you have curved feet.

Smooth soles, with maximum shock absorption are best for carpet on concrete surfaces, while good adhering tread stops slipping on smooth wooden surfaces.

Remember to have your shoes adjusted if you are predisposed to supination or pronation of the foot.

SPECIAL CONSIDERATIONS

No matter how safe the exercise programme, extra special care must be taken with people who have the following conditions.

PREGNANCY

Pregnancy causes increased arching of your lower back. Development of your abdominal muscles is essential to help counteract the strain on your vertebral column. Upper-body strength will significantly improve your posture.

Avoid flexibility work because your body releases the hormone Relaxin during pregnancy and it works to relax all the body's ligaments, creating high susceptibility to sprains and strains.

Do not exercise lying on your back after four months or the foetus weight may obstruct the blood flow back to your heart. Blockage of blood flow to the foetus may also occur.

Pregnant women also suffer more easily from overheating and low blood sugar levels.

There are many other potential problems for pregnant participants.

Consult qualified obstetric personnel before commencing your exercise programme.

Be aware that exercise may cause spontaneous abortion in the first three months of pregnancy.

OSTEOPOROSIS

Common in approximately 30% of post-menopausal women, osteoporosis is decreased bone mass which may lead to compression of vertebral bodies and bone fracture. Postural problems do occur.

The exact cause of Osteoporosis is still not known but research has shown that smoking, lack of calcium in your diet, inactivity, extreme thinness and oestrogen deficiencies are all contributing factors.

Exercise is important to help keep your bones strong. Walking is the best exercise but avoid rough terrain where you might fall.

Avoid twisting and turning quickly and consult your doctor and dietitian for hormonal and dietary advice.

SPECIAL NOTE: CHILDREN

Children are particularly at risk if they perform the dangerous exercises shown in this book. Their often weak but developing bodies may suffer irreversible damage if care is not taken.

The value of strength training during pre-adolescence remains a hotly debated issue. This age group is probably best suited to spending their time developing skills and cardio-vascular fitness.

Protect your children and make sure their teachers and coaches are not subjecting them to any dangerous exercises.

CHRONIC PROBLEMS

Diabetes, asthma, arthritis, obesity, high blood pressure and heart disease are chronic physical states that require you to receive a full medical clearance before you begin your exercise programme.

They should not stop you exercising but your programme will require some professional modification.

If you are recovering from injury, or illness, then you should seek a medical clearance and avoid strenuous exercise until you have fully recovered.